Infomedicine

Infomedicine

A CONSUMER'S GUIDE

TO THE LATEST

MEDICAL RESEARCH

FRED D. BALDWIN

AND

SUZANNE McINERNEY

LITTLE, BROWN AND COMPANY

BOSTON   NEW YORK   TORONTO   LONDON

FIRST EDITION

The author is grateful for permission to include the following previously copyrighted material:
"To CM: 55 YO WM w/CAD" by Joseph A. Gascho, M.D. Reprinted by permission of the author.
Excerpt from *The Official ABMS Directory of Board Certified Medical Specialists*, 1994, 26th edition. Published by Marquis Who's Who, a Reed Reference Publishing Company in cooperation with the American Board of Medical Specialists. Reprinted by permission of the publisher.

Library of Congress Cataloging-in-Publication Data

Baldwin, Fred D. (Fred Davis).
Infomedicine: a consumer's guide to the latest medical research /
by Fred D. Baldwin and Suzanne McInerney.
p.   cm.
Includes bibliographical references and index.
ISBN 0-316-07977-4 (hc)
ISBN 0-316-07910-3 (pb)
1. Medicine, Popular.   2. Consumer education.   3. Medicine—
Information services.   4. Health education.   5. Communication in
medicine.   I. McInerney, Suzanne.   II. Title.
RC81.B2335   1996
610—dc20   95-22146

10 9 8 7 6 5 4 3 2 1
MV-NY
Published simultaneously in Canada by Little, Brown & Company
(Canada) Limited

Printed in the United States of America

TO MY MOTHER, *Johanna Dyck Finke,*
who journeyed through life with enthusiasm,
wonder, and curiosity, and who—in her final
exploration—became the inspiration
for this book.
— S. M.

FOR MARILYN, *with love.*
— F. D. B.

Contents

Foreword

IF YOU ARE SERIOUSLY ILL, the odds are that — no matter what your income or education level — you will find yourself in the position where all of the basic life-or-death decisions are being made by people you scarcely know, with backgrounds you do not know at all, practicing in a facility whose track record in the management of your illness is also unknown to you.

You may be under the care of a well-meaning but unreflective doctor who routinely prescribes a "standard" treatment for each patient, without looking into the individual circumstances or the best treatment specifically for the patient. In some cases, you may even be under the care of physicians who have conflicts of interest — advancing their own careers through enrolling patients on research protocols, choosing treatments that generate higher fees, or, conversely, lowering costs for the managed health care system of which they are a part.

Where, in all these equations, would your own best medical interests as a patient fit in? I can't imagine just leaving my life, and the lives of my family, to the vagaries of an unevenly dependable health care system or to medical decisions made without my informed knowledge of the various treatment options.

For me, the greatest value of being a physician has come from having the tools to ensure that my own family and I receive the very best health care in times of illness.

Consider the following examples from my and my family's experience:

• My father-in-law is found to have prostate cancer, still in an early stage. His local doctors suggest radical prostatectomy. I (who have a good understanding of prostate cancer as a disease, the medical literature in general, and my father-in-law as an individual) am taken aback by the recommendation, which seems to ignore other important therapeutic options. I arrange his referral to a hospital more than a thousand miles away, where he can receive more appropriate treatment.

• I develop a fever of unknown origin. The physicians discuss aspirating joint fluid, lymph node biopsies, spinal taps, and liver studies. At least I know what these tests and their ramifications mean and can enter into a dialogue with the doctors.

• My mother develops breast cancer and requires a mastectomy, followed by postoperative adjuvant treatment by a medical oncologist. She belongs to a health maintenance organization, but I think that she could receive more appropriate treatment outside of her HMO. First, however, I have to convince her HMO that they should pay for the outside treatment — one that I consider to be medically justified.

In these situations, I was able to use my immediate medical knowledge, my knowledge of medical information sources, and my professional contacts to ensure that family members received the best possible care and, in each case, a favorable outcome. I was in a position to do it. Right now, most readers of this book are not.

The information age gives us consumer market journals if we want to research something as simple as buying a new toaster, or investment magazines and online computer resources if we want to purchase stock shares. The information age also makes medical information readily available, even if not in the "full disclosure" sense as other industries. Medical information of every kind and depth is available to anyone with the desire to use medical libraries, online resources reachable with a home computer, or institutions and patient organizations that provide many kinds of information.

The necessary digging may not always be easy, and time may frequently be of the essence. However, even in emergencies short of massive trauma or cardiac arrest, just being prepared to ask the right questions by being medically informed can often help you improve the situation. And in virtually any nonemergency contingency, possessing the most complete medical information possible can make a difference and — not uncommonly — a critical difference.

The authors of this book have provided a remarkably clear and practical "how-to manual," describing available tools for obtaining information necessary to find the best treatment and for using that information. Real-life stories of extraordinary patients illustrate the principles — and benefits — of becoming medically informed. The journey to the best treatment is not always easy, but it is one that can, and should, be undertaken by anyone with a serious illness and a desire to enjoy the best possible outcome.

LARRY M. WEISENTHAL, M.D., PH.D.
Associate Clinical Professor of Medicine,
University of California, Irvine
Medical Director, Weisenthal Cancer Group

How This Book Can Help You

IN THE SPRING of 1989, Suzanne McInerney, one of the authors of this book, sat beside her mother as her doctor told them that the results of a recent test given six months after surgery for colon cancer revealed the spread of cancer to her mother's liver. The two women listened as he outlined the possible courses of action: surgery, chemotherapy, or simply "waiting to see what happens."

When they met with her mother's oncologist, he explained that chemotherapy for this stage of colon cancer was a long shot and suggested that surgery would be the best choice. But the surgeon, they soon learned, would operate only if the tumor were confined to one area of the liver — something he couldn't be sure about until he operated. If he couldn't take out all the cancerous growth, the surgery would be a failure. Moreover, the operation itself was a massive insult to the body, weakening the system through blood loss and trauma — fatally, in far too many cases. Suzanne and her mother realized that "waiting to see what happens" meant passively accepting the inevitability of death, and that this was what the doctors regarded as the most humane and realistic option for a seventy-four-year-old woman.

Suzanne still recalls her own and her mother's sense of futility and helplessness. Her doctors, understandably, could think of her mother only as another luckless victim of metastatic colon cancer — one of thousands of cases each year. But to Suzanne, her mother's life, with its joys and sorrows and a million tender details, was inextricably entwined with Suzanne's own life, her husband's, and their children's. It was unacceptable to let her mother die without making every effort to find a way to save her.

Suzanne and her husband began finding out everything they could about treatments for advanced colon cancer. Fortunately, they had access to a medical library, where they could search for scientific literature on the most recent treatments in the field. Within a few days, they found journal articles by a surgeon who had devised a technique for removing tumors from the liver with a surgical mortality rate of zero and little blood loss and postoperative stress. Moreover, many of the surgeon's patients had survived at least five years beyond their operation — an unheard-of recovery rate with other types of surgery or chemotherapy treatment for this condition.

Suzanne and her husband were able to act upon that information and, with the support of their physicians, upon other information they subsequently found.

The result was that Suzanne's mother gained four additional years of life — *not* years as an invalid, with vital functions precariously maintained by machines and tubes, but four rich years. During these years, except for the two months before her death (not from cancer), she was able to live in complete independence and enjoy activities with her family. She took manifest pleasure from the knowledge that so many people — including, of course, Suzanne — had joined to make it possible for her to enjoy the gift of life.

Speaking of those years, Suzanne says: "They were especially rich years for me, too, because our relationship took on a whole new dimension. I rejoiced in her restored health and was grateful for the knowledge that I'd had a part in it. During that time, we became even closer than we'd been before."

The book you are reading began with Suzanne's experience. Subsequently, the authors talked to dozens of people who have made their own personal commitments to finding the best treatment for themselves or others they love and have acted on those commitments, sometimes with only modest gains, sometimes with spectacular success. What they have done, you can do.

In fact, the tools available to you today for your own search for the best treatment are far more sophisticated and effective than those Suzanne knew about, or that in some cases existed even as recently as a few years ago.

You cannot assume that your own doctor will necessarily know the best treatment for you. Advances in medical knowledge occur so fast that even the best-informed specialists can barely keep up with the literature in their fields. Unfortunately, you cannot even assume that your doctor will have mastered the information-finding tools described in this book. You, however, if you're willing to do some homework, can stay abreast of the work of the world's finest medical researchers, learn about clinical trials for new drugs, and exchange information with dozens of active patients like yourself. Armed with the knowledge you gain, determination, and a little luck, you can forge a working partnership with your physician that will make both of you far more effective than either of you could be alone.

This book is strictly about finding and using medical information. It contains no health tips, no recommendations on treatment, no endorsement of products or services, and, above all, no promise of quick cures or ready-made miracles. Its authors understand that all serious illness is frightening, that technical literature can make difficult reading, that human judgment is fallible, and that sometimes the best you can hope for is improving your chances of success. But we also affirm that reliable knowledge can help you avoid unnecessary surgery and suffering, locate lifesaving drugs, and, even in the face of the most dangerous illnesses, often prevail against odds that your doctor may think are hopeless.

One section of this book focuses on the use of personal computers in locating the best treatment. You can benefit from this material even if you have no prior computer experience. Even if you have never dreamed of logging on to an online information service, you can recognize (and make sure your doctor realizes) what truly amazing medical resources you can bring into your own home over ordinary telephone lines from the Internet and other sources — both documentary information and advice from people who care. Perhaps you'll decide that computers are easier to use than you may have supposed.

Whether the problem you face is life-threatening, like cancer, or slowly disabling, like rheumatoid arthritis, the research techniques explained here can guide you to treatment possibilities your busy doctor might otherwise overlook. Yet this book is more than a list of state-of-the-art medical information resources; it also explains how to use information to become an active partner with your doctor.

The principles and techniques you'll learn here have been proved in practice by courageous patients with no formal medical training. They educated themselves and made tough personal decisions. Some of them had to contend not only with physical illness but with the negative attitudes of physicians who knew less about recent medical literature than they did. You'll read their stories: two parents whose persistence saved their son from blindness, a woman whose stubborn search for usable answers saved herself from disfiguring surgery, a man whose efforts saved a family member's life, and many others.

"The reward," Suzanne says, speaking of her own experience, "was worth every bit of effort all of us put into it. But the battle would have been lost before it was ever begun if we hadn't seized on that glimmer of opportunity in the stacks of the medical library."

You don't have to settle for anything less than the best treatment for yourself or someone you love. Please don't settle for less.

Acknowledgments

A COMPLETE LIST of all the people who have helped with this book would require at least a full chapter. They include medical librarians, staff members of public and private health care organizations, representatives of medical associations and patient advocacy groups, information professionals, and scores, if not hundreds, of individual patients and physicians who have communicated with the authors in person, by telephone, through CompuServe forums, and on the Internet. We are grateful both for their patience and for their demonstrated enthusiasm for making reliable medical information available to the widest possible audience.

We are especially grateful to the courageous men and women who permitted us to tell their stories in these pages. Some, whose full names are used, are identified by their real names; others by assumed first names. To each of them, we offer our heartfelt thanks for teaching and inspiring us by their example.

We are indebted to the medical reference librarians who shared their knowledge and skills. A few of the many who helped us immeasurably are Eric P. Delozier and Sandra Wood, George T. Harrell Library, the Pennsylvania State University College of

Medicine; Judy F. Welch, Carlisle (Pennsylvania) Hospital Medical Library; Elizabeth Coldsmith, Harrisburg (Pennsylvania) Hospital Medical Library Services; Susan Robeshaw, Geisinger Medical Center Library; and Judith Logan, Lyman Maynard Stowe Library, University of Connecticut Health Center.

In addition, we thank the many staff members of the National Library of Medicine, especially Sheldon Kotzin, Robert Mehnert, and Carolyn Tilley, who not only answered questions but made available the illustrations of NLM print and online resources that appear in this book. Thanks are due also to Ann Paietta, National Network of Libraries of Medicine, New York Academy of Medicine.

For their valuable comments and suggestions on various portions of the manuscript, we thank E. Andrew Balas, M.D.; Noel Ballentine, M.D.; Loren Buhle, Ph.D.; Leslie Carr, R.N.; K. Danner Clouser, Ph.D.; Ian Gilchrist, M.D.; Edward Del Grosso, M.D.; Robert Dye, M.D.; Alan S. Goldberg, Esq.; Lee Hancock, Ph.D.; Ann Kerwin, Ph.D.; Lauren Dieguez Langford; Roseanna Lenker, R.N.; Edward Madara; Gary Malet, M.D.; Barbara Quint; John Ross; Eugene P. Schonfeld, Ph.D.; and David Weisenthal.

To Robert H. Bonneau, Ph.D., the Pennsylvania State University College of Medicine, Department of Microbiology and Immunology, we are indebted for his encouragement, advice on numerous sections of the manuscript, and instruction in the complex field of psychoneuroimmunology. Also, for providing extensive background material through numerous interviews, we wish to thank Robert Zelis, M.D., Division of Cardiology, Department of Medicine, also at the Pennsylvania State University College of Medicine.

Our deep appreciation goes to Jennifer Josephy of Little, Brown, for her early enthusiasm for this book. Special thanks must go to our editor, Geoffrey Kloske, for his adroit professional advice and for his optimism; to Betty Power, for her most valuable copyediting contribution; and to our literary agent, Richard Balkin, who championed our cause and brought his good cheer to the project.

Finally, we acknowledge our deepest gratitude to our spouses, Marilyn H. Keener and Joseph J. McInerney, whose love and support sustained us.

PART I

YOU CAN

MAKE YOUR OWN

DECISIONS

You can and should become an active partner with your doctor in crucial health decisions. Knowing how to find and use state-of-the-art medical information is the key. No one, including the most competent and dedicated physicians, can keep up with today's explosive growth in medical knowledge — much of it compiled in approximately 380,000 articles per year. You can, however, find and master the information you need to get the best available treatment, including possibilities your doctor may not have mentioned. Evidence from many determined patients proves the value of seeking out the latest medical research. You can learn to do what they did, whether on your own behalf or that of someone you love.

1.

You Can't Ask Too
Many Questions

GAYLE ALLISON WASN'T sure whether the doctor standing before her was the twelfth or the fifteenth she'd consulted. After ten years of illness and consultations in several different cities, it was easy to lose count. She does, however, remember quite clearly what he told her.

"He stood there," she says, "and said, 'Look, Gayle! There's nothing wrong with you!' "

He wasn't the first doctor to tell her that. Her problems had begun with a ringing in her right ear that got worse and worse until she had almost no hearing on that side. She experienced headaches and, in time, dizziness and nausea. X-rays of her stomach and spine revealed no organic problems. Accepting the possibility (suggested by more than one doctor) that her symptoms might be psychosomatic, Gayle even consulted a psychiatrist to be sure that her symptoms were not imaginary.

In the late 1980s, Gayle went to a new clinic to consult an ear, nose, and throat specialist whom she hadn't previously consulted. He listened to her symptoms and suggested a magnetic resonance imaging (MRI) scan "to rule out the possibility of a tumor." (Although X-rays of the abdomen and elsewhere had been ordered for Gayle when she complained of nausea, she'd never been X-rayed above her neck.)

The MRI revealed that Gayle did have a tumor — something called an acoustic neuroma. An acoustic neuroma grows on the cranial nerve that controls hearing and balance. After a decade of being told that nothing was wrong with her, it was actually a relief to Gayle to hear that at least she'd been right all along about her symptoms. The specialist explained to her that an acoustic neuroma is both benign (meaning that it does not spread to other organs) and surgically removable.

But she also learned dismaying news. First, an acoustic neuroma, although not malignant, is dangerous. Its slow, inexorable growth within a bony cavity behind the inner ear squeezes nerves against bone. This leads to the kinds of symptoms that Gayle experienced, and these symptoms become more severe as the tumor grows. If left to grow unchecked, the tumor may crush the nerves that control digestion and breathing — causing death.

Second, the textbook approaches for surgical removal of an acoustic neuroma all carry considerable risk to the patient. The operation is delicate and requires extraordinary surgical skill. The surgeon must slice away at the tumor within a small, irregularly shaped space through which many nerves connect to the brain. Depending largely on the size of the tumor, which can range from that of a pea to larger than a walnut, the operation to remove it can take from six to over twenty hours.

The risk isn't to life; almost no one dies from acoustic neuroma surgery. But once the tumor has reached a certain size, it is nearly impossible for the surgeon to avoid damage, both to the nerve on which the tumor itself is growing and to other nerves pressing against it. A high percentage of the survivors of acoustic neuroma surgery emerge from anesthesia to discover that they can no longer control muscles on one side of the face. Their smiles are twisted, their speech slurred, and it may be months before they can chew without dribbling food from one side of the mouth. If they're very unlucky, they may stagger as they walk. In many cases, their insurance companies automatically consider them eligible for full disability payments.

The doctor who accurately diagnosed Gayle's condition told her that she had little real choice. She was in no immediate danger; acoustic neuromas grow slowly. But, he told her, the severity of her symptoms suggested that surgery should be performed sooner rather than later.

AN AGGRESSIVE SEARCH FOR TREATMENT OPTIONS

If Gayle had learned one thing in nine years, however, it was that doctors are sometimes wrong. She started reading about the probable effects of surgical removal of her tumor and decided that she didn't want any part of that. One brochure she read gave the name of a national self-help group, the Acoustic Neuroma Association. She called its offices and, although she received encouragement, was told that her doctor was probably right. Was there no alternative to surgery? she asked. Well, she was told, almost as an afterthought, there was one alternative — something called a "gamma knife."

Persisting and probing, Gayle learned that the gamma knife involves focusing high-intensity radiation on a small tumor, hopefully killing it in place. The tumor doesn't vanish, but, if the operation is successful, it seems to shrivel up like a grape turning into a raisin. Except for severe but temporary headaches, there are seldom adverse side effects. The technique isn't always successful, but the risks seemed to Gayle to be far lower than those associated with conventional surgery. Besides, even if the tumor didn't die, surgery remained as a last resort.

Ironically, the specialist who had accurately diagnosed her condition strongly opposed her choice of treatment. He pointed out (correctly) that the gamma knife was not the standard mode of treatment for acoustic neuromas. Gayle showed him the journal articles she'd collected that seemed to indicate that radiosurgery (gamma knife is a radiosurgical technique) offered significant advantages over the "standard" approach. She recalls that he refused to read them and became angry at her persistence.

Nevertheless, on July 26, 1988, Gayle entered Presbyterian University Hospital in Pittsburgh, then the only hospital in the

United States in which gamma knife surgery was performed. She sat in a chair while technicians immobilized her head inside a device resembling a cross between a science-fiction space jockey's headset and a beauty-shop hair dryer. ("I describe it to people as a huge football helmet," she says.) Using magnetic resonance imaging to locate the tumor accurately, the doctors destroyed it with precisely focused radiation.

Gayle says it took her three years to recover completely, but recover she did. After five years, the usual time for evaluating the ultimate success of tumor surgery, her tests show no evidence of tumor growth and no complications.

"You can never ask too many questions," Gayle says in summing up her experience. "If a doctor becomes insulted [by questions], you'd better look for another doctor."

THE CRUCIAL DECISIONS ARE UP TO YOU

Eventually, Gayle not only received a correct diagnosis but was able to take advantage of a treatment that left her with no damaging side effects. Her commitment to be an active patient — her stubbornness, if you will — exemplifies the attitude that may be required to make your own efforts a success. This chapter will tell you why you need to make that same commitment, even if you are luckier in your physicians than Gayle often was.

The central thesis of this book is simple: *you and your doctor, working together, will make better decisions than either of you could make alone.* Your goal should be a partnership based on your physicians' expertise and a shared respect for your ultimate right to make crucial decisions for yourself.

Of course, for as long as you've been an adult, you've been responsible for your own decisions. At a purely logical level, you know this. You know, for example, that you can't be compelled to undergo surgery, any more than you can be compelled to floss your teeth every day. If you're ever scheduled for surgery, the release form you'll be asked to sign will state quite clearly that the decision to accept the risk is your responsibility. This point may seem too obvious to state, except that, faced with serious medical decisions, we tend forget it.

WHY YOUR DOCTOR MAY NOT "KNOW BEST"

From time to time, "medical miracles" make headlines. If a team of researchers discovers a cure for AIDS, you can be sure you'll be bombarded with stories about it. But for every highly publicized medical breakthrough, there are dozens — thousands, actually — of less spectacular advances that materially improve the quality of medical care and thus improve someone's chances of recovery from a dangerous medical condition.

The true breakthrough for you may not be a celebrated "miracle cure" but something that simply tilts the odds a bit more in your favor.

For example, finding the most effective chemotherapy for a given form of cancer can sometimes be tricky, because not all people respond to a treatment in the same way, even if they have an identical form of the disease.

Scientists have devised a chemotherapeutic testing procedure (often called "chemosensitivity testing" or "cancer drug resistance testing") using a patient's cells outside his or her body to predetermine which agents will be effective. This new procedure, which was first reported in the medical research literature long before it was reported in the popular press, demonstrated that drugs identified as active in the laboratory were seven times more likely to be effective against cancers in a particular patient. Early knowledge of this test procedure could obviously have a major impact on a cancer patient's chance of survival.

You can't really expect your doctor to become aware of all research literature as soon as it is published. Several thousand medical journals are published in English, not to mention those in other languages, and no one can ever read more than a tiny fraction of them. Altogether, the National Library of Medicine adds more than 380,000 new citations each year to its medical databases.

The importance of this for you is suggested by studies of the differences in drugs prescribed by physicians in general practice and those who are research oriented. For example, a recent study by Dr. Elliott Antman, Harvard Medical School, shows that common aspirin — almost universally accepted as useful for patients who have had heart attacks — was prescribed by only about 53 percent of personal physicians; however, research-oriented cardiologists prescribed it for 84 percent of their patients. By contrast, calcium-channel blockers, a class of heart attack drugs believed in the 1980s to be extremely promising, have not proved as effective as hoped in clinical trials. But in 1990, Dr. Antman found that 49 percent of nonresearch doctors continued to prescribe them; only 17 percent of research-oriented doctors did.

Bear in mind that being a "specialist," meaning a physician with a recognized medical specialty, is not necessarily the same thing as being research-oriented. Outside of academic medicine, where research is often required for promotion and where new treatments are constantly discussed, not even specialists can be expected to keep up with everything in their own fields. Can you feel sure that your busy cardiologist will have read the eighty to one hundred articles that appear every four or five weeks in *American Journal of Cardiology, Journal of American College of Cardiology, American Heart Journal, British Heart Journal,* and *Progress on Cardiovascular Diseases,* to mention only five of the better-known journals among many that report on treatments for heart disease?

Finally, if keeping up with the state of medical knowledge is a problem for specialists, think of what it means for your family doctor. He or she, whether a solo practitioner or a member of a group practice or outpatient clinic, is a busy person. Doctors not only have patients with many different kinds of problems, but they are also inundated by nonmedical paperwork. Nonclinical journals and magazines written for physician audiences regularly carry articles on coping with insurance forms, governmental regulations, and the dangers of physician burnout from overwork.

A series of articles that appeared during 1993 and 1994 in the *Journal of the American Medical Association* encouraged physicians to use the computerized databases discussed in this book as tools in their clinical practice. The articles instructed doctors in the use of software programs such as "Grateful Med" (described in chapter 11).

Unfortunately, you can't assume that your physician will take the time to do this kind of computer-assisted literature search, knows how to do it, or feels the need to do it. A spokesperson for the National Library of Medicine recently estimated that "fewer than 20 percent" of the nation's physicians had ever done an online search. Of course, some doctors may ask hospital librarians to do searches for them. Even so, the computer-literate physicians who participate regularly in the online discussion groups described in chapter 12 conjecture that the NLM official's estimate is likely to be tactfully high. ("It's a *lot* fewer," one doctor wrote.)

YOUR DOCTOR MAY NOT MENTION ALL YOUR OPTIONS

It's important not only to appreciate Gayle Allison's courage and stubbornness but also to understand why her specialist thought that she was making a serious mistake and even became angry over her refusal to take his advice. You may be thinking, "My doctor would never be like that!" Perhaps not, but the reactions she encountered can't be dismissed as the odd personal prejudices of the physicians she happened to consult.

Joseph Anderson can offer insights on this issue. Joseph works for an organization that monitors hospital accreditation standards. He's completing a doctoral dissertation on the education of professionals. He also has three things in common with Allison: he's lived with the symptoms of an acoustic neuroma, chose the gamma knife option to destroy the tumor, and chose this option *against* the advice of someone he considers a very competent neurosurgeon. For both professional and personal reasons, he's given a lot of thought to why members of the medical profession may be slow to embrace a treatment that seems to have much to recommend it, compared to conventional surgery.

One reason, Joseph explains, is that it's possible to make a very good case for medical conservatism. Medical history is filled with stories of "miracle" cures that weren't — drugs with adverse side effects, and so on. Doctors, particularly those who deal with tumors (malignant or otherwise) are trained to look at long-term results. However promising drugs may seem during clinical trials to evaluate their effectiveness, no one can guarantee that problems will not come to light later.

That experts may disagree about the best approach to a problem should come as no surprise. The important question is why

Joseph's neurosurgeon did not even mention the radiosurgery option until Joseph pressed hard with questions.

That question leads Joseph to comment on attitudes rooted in the nature of medical specialization. Neurosurgeons, he notes, stand near the peak of the medical profession where prestige is concerned — and rightly so, because of the skill their practice requires. When they see a tumor and know that it's operable, their instinct is to operate.

Similar attitudes exist within other medical specialties. For example, national rates of radical prostatectomies (surgical removal of the prostate gland) increased almost sixfold between 1984 and 1990. This increase occurred because blood tests had improved detection of prostate cancers at an early stage, and radical prostatectomy was the most commonly prescribed treatment for such tumors. Since more were being found, more were being removed. There is currently a debate within the medical profession as to when radical prostatectomies should be the treatment of choice, but the increase in such surgery occurred before clinical evidence could be considered to have demonstrated that it was warranted. Critics of "standard" practices contend that specialists trained to perform one procedure may not look at other procedures objectively; that is, "When your only tool is a hammer, you see every problem as a nail."

Although physicians associated with teaching and research facilities are most likely to know of new medical advances, they will not necessarily recommend them to patients. They may wait until the value of a treatment has been demonstrated beyond all reasonable doubt in large, randomized clinical trials, ignoring the accumulated, although not conclusive, evidence gathered bit by bit in smaller case studies.

Moreover, medicine, like other fields, is characterized by patterns of behavior that vary not only over time but from place to place. A physician's sense of what is meant by "standard" treatment may be a function of what other physicians in the immediate geographical area are doing. The U.S. Office of Technology Assessment (OTA), which studies policy issues for the Congress, analyzed medical literature through the early 1980s and found large differences in surgical and other procedures across geographic areas. For example, hysterectomy rates varied fivefold across hospital service areas within the province of Manitoba, Canada. Large variations across states were found for other procedures such as hernia repairs, appendectomies, and cesarean sections. Within one state, rates of hospitalization for back injury varied *tenfold* across hospital service areas. For you, this means that getting a second opinion from a physician in your immediate area, as important as that may be, does not necessarily guarantee that you will get a significantly more comprehensive perspective. A second opinion is desirable but definitely not a substitute for learning as much as possible on your own about your treatment options.

YOU NEED TO *SAY* YOU WANT TO BE AN ACTIVE PARTNER

Many physicians do not discuss options fully because they feel that patients do not want to confront difficult choices. The active patients interviewed for this book frequently expressed resentment of this attitude, even while acknowledging that it might be well intended.

It's understandable that physicians are often influenced by their patients' real or apparent longing for simple, immediate answers. Patients may signal by their manner, or imply by their silence, that they expect their doctor to know and decide what's "best." Even Joseph Anderson, normally inclined to ask questions, admits that his first reaction to being told that he had a kind of brain tumor was to want it out at once.

"I wanted surgery," he says. "I wanted to get rid of this thing. I wasn't a rational person."

In the end, Joseph forced himself to ask questions and, like Gayle Allison, he's glad he did.

He ticks off the benefits of his decision. The whole process cost roughly one-third the cost of conventional acoustic neuroma surgery, a ratio that he says still prevails. He lost only three days of work, compared to months for most acoustic neuroma survivors (those who are not permanently disabled). Most important, of course, he's healthy and physically fit.

Physicians debate among themselves how much information a "typical" patient wants and can use effectively. You need not be concerned with what someone else may want, so long as you can communicate the message that *you*, typical or not, want to learn as much as possible about your condition and its treatment and that you are willing to listen carefully and read as necessary. If you don't do that, your physicians may assume that you expect them to screen your options for you. In short, if you want to be informed of all your choices, you have a responsibility to make that fact crystal clear.

YOUR GOAL IS A WORKING PARTNERSHIP

There's nothing scandalous in the notion that the physicians you consult may *not* "know best," nor should you be surprised that physicians, like all of us, are vulnerable to both personal and professional biases. These are simply factors to take into account if you want the best treatment for yourself and those you care about.

Moreover, as this book will repeatedly emphasize, the kind of treatment you get from doctors is also very much a function of your own knowledge, your own attitudes, and your own recognition of the limitations and pressures under which doctors are forced to function. Medical decisions are often difficult. Stephen R. Covey, in his best-selling personal development guide *The Seven Habits of Highly Effective People*, urges, "Seek first to understand, then to be understood." Your life may depend on how well your doctors understand you and your needs; that's more likely to happen when you understand how hard it is for them to keep up with medical knowledge, as well as the subtle and not-so-subtle factors that may cause them to volunteer less information than it is in your interests to have.

Fortunately, many physicians embody the intellectual humility expressed by the late Lewis Thomas, M.D., whose graceful essays on medical and scientific topics have become classics. Thomas wrote the following lines as a preface to *Cecil Textbook of Medicine*, a standard text in internal medicine:

> The greatest discovery in this most productive of centuries has been the discovery that we are profoundly ignorant. We

know very little about the human body, and we understand even less. I wish there were some formal courses somewhere on medical ignorance, and textbooks as well, although they would have to be very heavy volumes.

This passage has inspired a unique curriculum called "medical ignorance" at the medical school of the University of Arizona. Students there are required to do research, even if they do not plan research careers, to remind them of how much remains to be learned in medicine. They also are taught to evaluate their own beliefs against a six-variety classification of "ignorance." The categories range from simple lack of knowledge (recognized as such) to far more dangerous problems, including erroneous beliefs (not recognized as such). The philosophy underlying this course is a good prescription for doctors and patients alike.

Your primary care physician and most of the specialists you encounter may be knowledgeable and experienced. Even so, you can never be certain that the treatment they will suggest is the best medical science has to offer.

Your doctor must attempt to meet the needs of hundreds of patients. But you have only one body, one life. You alone have everything at stake in the outcome of your case. It may be that you can safely assume your doctor knows best, but you shouldn't bet your life on it.

For *your* medical problem — whether common or rare — you of course have no guarantee that there exists some thoroughly tested new drug or technique that your doctor hasn't mentioned. Even if there is, its advantages may not seem as compelling to you as the advantages of gamma knife surgery seemed to Gayle Allison and to Joseph Anderson, or as the innovative approach to liver surgery proved to be in the case of Suzanne's mother. The most thorough search imaginable may yield only the satisfaction of knowing that you explored every avenue you could think of. That's no small benefit in itself, of course, particularly if you're doing the exploration for someone you care about. Choosing not to explore is itself a choice — one that could deny you or someone you love the knowledge of a lifesaving or life-enhancing discovery.

2.

How Information Pays Off

GARY SCHINE, A small-business consultant who lives in Providence, Rhode Island, says that he didn't get nervous at all until the oncologist "started talking about bone marrow." Gary, then only thirty-eight years old, had simply thought himself a bit out of shape, although climbing two flights of stairs left him exhausted.

When the results of bone marrow tests came back, the oncologist tried to be as gentle as possible, but the news was devastating. "All he knew," Gary says, "was that it was some kind of leukemia. He didn't know what form it was. He didn't know whether I had months or weeks to live. His parting words were, 'Make sure your life insurance is paid up and your health insurance is paid up.'"

Two weeks later, Gary received some slight encouragement. His disease was hairy-cell leukemia (HCL), a rare form of leukemia that develops slowly. The oncologist explained that a splenectomy (surgical removal of the spleen) might give him several years of relatively normal life and that chemotherapy might then slow the disease further. Gary would experience flu-like symptoms and loss of mental concentration as side effects of the drugs. With luck, he might live as much as ten years, long enough to see his two young children reach their teens. "But," Gary says, "he was very clear on the fact that there was no cure for it."

Gary decided to do his own research. He called a local chapter of the Leukemia Society of America, learned that a clinical trial of a new treatment for HCL was in progress, and used his computer to locate more information on the trial. What he found seemed almost too good to be true.

"Three months before my diagnosis," he says, "the *New England Journal of Medicine* had an article about a new drug that was then in clinical trial. Although only twelve people with this kind of leukemia were being reported on in that article, eleven of them were in complete remission, and one was in partial remission. It just stunned me that I could be told one thing by an oncologist and read this article that told me quite a different story. I figured that without a scientific background I must be misinterpreting it. I took it across the street to a doctor friend of mine who said, 'No, you're not misinterpreting this at all. This is wonderful!' "

The oncologist who had diagnosed him tried to discourage him from pursuing an "experimental" therapy. Gary persisted. He chose a trial then underway in California and, after a few rough weeks of temporary reactions to the new drug, began to feel better. Within two months, he was working full time again and "exercising for the first time in ten years."

Today, four years later, Gary is free of all HCL symptoms and, as far as he or anyone else can determine, is completely cured of leukemia. He still works hard as a business consultant. He's also written a book on his experience entitled *If the President Had Cancer*. But his life has also changed somewhat — very much for the better. On most days he runs between two and three miles, and he says that he makes a point of spending more time with his family.

Gary's story shows how risky it can be to assume that a physician, even a specialist, will know about the latest medical research. He took the first step, one that led to his complete recovery, by not accepting his doctor's prognosis that his disease was incurable *and* by deciding to learn for himself all he could about every possible treatment option. Gary discovered the existence of a highly promising course of treatment almost immediately. But his experience in finding a solid lead so quickly isn't necessarily typical.

PERSISTENCE PAYS OFF

In fact, the search for a successful treatment may go on for years. That's the way it was for Yasmin and her husband, Jamshed, both of whose ancestors come from present-day Iran. That genetic heritage was significant, but they had no way of knowing its relevance when, in the late 1970s, their fourteen-year-old son, Karl, began losing vision in his right eye.

After Karl had spent months following a futile regimen of eye exercises suggested by an optometrist, Yasmin took him to an ophthalmologist, who correctly diagnosed his problem as Behçet's syndrome, a hereditary disease that can attack various parts of the body, including the retina of the eye. The ophthalmologist prescribed steroids and cortisone injections, but these treatments weren't working. Finally, a friend arranged for Yasmin and Jamshed to visit the late Robert Mendelsohn, M.D., a doctor who believed so strongly in patient empowerment that he was then considered a radical within the medical profession.

Dr. Mendelsohn began by admitting his own ignorance: all he knew about Behçet's syndrome was a few vague memories from medical school.

"When I don't know a great deal about a disease," he told Yasmin and Jamshed, "I open a medical encyclopedia and see who has written a definitive description. If they're good enough to write the definitive description in the encyclopedia, they're good enough to look at your child."

Dr. Mendelsohn had three references open. But he hadn't contacted any of these experts himself.

"The first thing you do," he continued, "*you* should call these people up, one by one. And *you* talk to them. Also, you tell me that your son is taking steroids. You need to know what steroids do. You need to be far more educated than you are in *everything* this child takes."

"Basically," Yasmin sums up, "he told me that *I* had to do it all. He told us, 'Assume control. Interrogate your doctors. Make decisions. Take choices into your own hands.' "

The couple had paid Dr. Mendelsohn a substantial fee for this consultation. Yasmin recalls:

"I went out of the office thinking, 'I've been had!' I was so angry that *he* didn't do what I wanted him to do that I kind of did nothing for about another month. At which point my son started losing vision in his left eye. That jolted me."

At last Yasmin and Jamshed committed themselves to a search process that was to stretch across several years.

They began by searching the medical literature in a university teaching hospital library. They learned that Behçet's syndrome, although rare, most often occurs within ethnic groups whose members seldom marry outside the group. Its frequency is highest in Japan and some Middle Eastern cultures.

They also began a search for expertise. None of the entries in Dr. Mendelsohn's medical encyclopedias had been written by an ophthalmologist. Two were by immunologists, one by a rheumatologist. One of these experts referred them to a student of his, already becoming eminent, who was getting good results with Behçet's syndrome from a process that involved transferring white blood cells from a healthy donor carrying the problematic gene. A literature search at a medical school library also revealed that Behçet's syndrome was treatable with a drug used in cancer therapy. Its success rate was excellent, but its potential side effects were disturbing.

Yasmin, who had once been afraid of questioning doctors, grew bolder with practice. At one point, like the director of a small medical task force, she was coordinating communications among five physicians in five different cities: the ophthalmologist, the rheumatologist, an infectious disease specialist, their son's original pediatrician, and Dr. Mendelsohn, whom she continued to consult on how to ask questions. She saw to it that every one of these doctors received copies of everything that any one of them discovered or suggested, and she kept copies for herself and Jamshed. Using the research skills that had once earned her a Ph.D. in literature but that she had never imagined applying to medicine, she also made contacts with experts in Israel and Japan.

After much thought and study, the two parents decided to go with the blood replacement therapy, using Jamshed as the donor. For some time this led to almost miraculous results: Karl's vision improved from 20/400 to 20/40. He graduated from high school.

In college, however, his vision began to deteriorate again, and the family decided to go with the cancer drug.

The chemotherapy went on for thirteen weeks.

"Finally," Yasmin says, "my husband and son walked in one day — I'll never forget it — and Jamshed said, 'Karl doesn't have it anymore.' "

Today Karl is a healthy adult employed by a high-tech firm, his eyesight only moderately impaired. Looking back on the experience, Yasmin's only regret is that she and Jamshed didn't take charge sooner.

"I'd gone in [to Dr. Mendelsohn] with the same notion I'd brought to every other doctor," she says. "I was going to walk in, and he was going to tell us how we could save our child, and everything was going to be all right. And it seemed that he hadn't. But he had!"

This family's experience shows the value of persistence. The search for a cure for Karl's illness stretched across several years, but it was ultimately successful. It also shows how the patient-doctor relationship can evolve over time. By the end of the process, Yasmin had effectively become general manager of a project to save her son's eyesight and, like any good manager, had learned to mobilize the knowledge and command the respect of team members whose technical qualifications far exceeded her own. The model of a nontechnical manager directing the work of specialists is common in business and industry. It's a model that requires a manager to learn a technical vocabulary, and that can't be done overnight. Once it's working, however, it can be highly productive.

GETTING YOURSELF TAKEN SERIOUSLY

Sometimes, of course, the problem is that doctors don't give your problem their best attention. Consider now a story from Joanne Goldberg, who lives in Boston.

About two years after receiving silicone-gel implants following breast cancer surgery, Joanne began experiencing pain in her joints and muscles along with other symptoms. But her doctors didn't take her very seriously, even when she told them she could no longer tie the laces of her walking shoes. After ordering tests and pronouncing the results "normal," her doctor prescribed a nonsteroidal anti-inflammatory drug. He suggested no further diagnostic measures.

Joanne decided to look up the drug in a reference book and learned that rheumatoid arthritis is one of the conditions for which it is prescribed. Next, by studying the *Merck Manual of Diagnosis and Therapy* (described in chapter 5), she learned that symptoms resembling those of rheumatoid arthritis may involve the immune system's response to presences the body regards as foreign. Might her symptoms, she wondered, be caused by her silicone implants?

About that time, Joanne started using CompuServe, a commercial online information service. ("Online" means that these services are accessible by a personal computer linked to a telephone.) She logged on to a health-related database and typed in a single word: "silicone." Back came a raft of citations from medical journals. They had titles like "Tissue Reactions to Breast Implants Coated with Polyurethane," "Post-Mammoplasty Connective Tissue Disease," and "Silicone and Rheumatic Disease." All were in mainstream medical journals, spanning a period of almost thirty years. The articles she secured confirmed that her symptoms might well be related to silicone. Her husband, too, joined in her search and spent many hours helping her locate additional material.

Armed with her new information, Joanne sought out second and third opinions. The responses were very different from the near-dismissals she'd received earlier. "In the eyes of the practitioners," she says, "this bibliography seemed somehow to move me from the stuff of which 'Oprah' is made to a subject worthy of further consideration and clinical investigation." A surgeon read her material and agreed it was highly likely that the implants were the cause of her symptoms. She underwent surgery for their removal. Her aching joints and other symptoms soon subsided, then disappeared.

Joanne's experience testifies to how information, careful reasoning, and personal tenacity in presenting one's case can win the credibility that will almost always earn a physician's close attention. She and her husband were able to locate the information they needed by pursuing the task together. Like many others, she learned that when you can't do everything for yourself, other ways may open.

WITH A LITTLE HELP FROM HER FRIENDS

Laurel Simmons's journey to Seattle, where she would undergo a bone marrow transplant, did not begin at Boston's Logan Airport on the day of her departure. It began in 1987 when she was diagnosed with leukemia, one day after her twenty-fifth birthday.

Laurel, a manager at a computer science laboratory at the Massachusetts Institute of Technology (MIT), did what seemed natural to her. She talked openly about her illness.

"As soon as I was diagnosed," recalls Laurel, "I started telling as many people as I could. It was a spontaneous thing — not a decision I made. We work in an environment in which problems are solved by gathering the necessary information and working hard at the solution. The idea of powerlessness is very foreign to many of my friends."

Laurel's friends provided a kind of support that her family, who also did everything they could, were too stunned emotionally to provide. Information gathering was as natural to them as breathing. They scoured libraries and, like some *Mission Impossible* task force, met for collective problem solving.

"Our group even had a name," Laurel says, "after the name of a beloved grandfather of one of its members. During meetings, I mostly sat there while everyone went about the business of figuring out what needed to be done."

Laurel herself became a student of her disease, poring over all the materials on chronic myelogenous leukemia (CML) that her friends had gathered for her. Her first oncologist seemed to resent her persistent questions. She came to feel that he was being less than candid with her, and she lost confidence in him.

"Everyone insisted that we find a new oncologist," she says. "I was terrified. It's a very hard and scary thing to terminate a relationship with a doctor. There is a lot of fear that if you reject a doctor you will not be cared for anymore. It's a tough hurdle to get over."

Laurel did, however, find a new oncologist, and this time the chemistry was right.

" 'I absolutely have to have the truth,' " she recalls telling him. "Despite the fact that I was angry and nervous, he took it quite well and said something like, 'No problem.' And it wasn't. I have known him for seven years, and he has always been totally honest with me and respectful of my intelligence and my need to know details."

Her first oncologist had recommended a bone marrow transplant and suggested the Fred Hutchinson Cancer Research Center in Seattle, Washington. Her new oncologist seconded both recommendations, and Laurel's team followed up. While one friend found information on transplants, another checked out the Fred Hutchinson Center, verifying that it has a world-class reputation. Others became fund-raisers to defray costs beyond those that her insurance would cover. Still others researched living accommodations in Seattle and, Laurel recalls gratefully, "took on the task of managing my daily life." Someone persuaded a major airline to donate ten round-trip tickets, so that at least one member of the team could be with her during her entire stay there. Team members even foresaw *their own* need for emotional support and planned to back each other up at especially difficult times.

In one form of bone marrow transplant, the patient's own bone marrow is extracted, "cleaned," and restored to the body. In other instances, the malignant blood cells within the patient's own bone marrow are killed by a combination of radiation and drugs, and the patient receives fresh marrow from a healthy donor whose blood chemistry matches the patient's as nearly as possible. Laurel needed a donor, and all three of her brothers offered blood for testing. The blood sample from one of them, Stuart, proved a near-perfect match, so he joined her in Seattle.

The Fred Hutchinson Center proved to be as excellent as its reputation. Although Laurel was hospitalized for 40 days and was an outpatient in Seattle for 25 days after that, the procedure went well. Returning home in late 1987, she was back at work by the following spring.

In 1990, Laurel's cancer returned. Because of certain physical complications, she was unable to have a second transplant, but — again after careful research — she located (in Boston) an innovative therapy that has kept her leukemia in remission for well over three years now. That's long enough to make her prospects promising, whatever uncertainties remain.

"It was a kind of hell at the time," Laurel says, groping for words, "but the physical pain disappears from your memory. But the emotional side . . . I wish it had never happened, there's no question about that, but I have a lot of good experiences to focus on. I was so supported and so loved and always thought I was in such good hands."

Laurel's experience shows not only the value of information but the value of using all of your resources in a time of serious illness — including, of course, friends. Few people have friends and colleagues as skilled as Laurel's in searching for information, but many people have friends and family who can help with specific tasks. Becoming an active patient may involve thinking through a complex process. One element of that process is finding ways to free your time and energy for doing what you most need to do and learning what you most need to learn.

MORE OPTIONS THAN YOUR DOCTOR KNOWS

Here's one more example of the value of absolutely up-to-date medical information combined with a determination to see it put to use. Al Musella is a podiatrist. His four years of postgraduate medical training in diagnosing and treating disorders of the feet had taught him nothing about brain tumors. Nevertheless, his search for the best treatment for a family member named Janet led him to medical literature that eminent cancer specialists in his area had never seen.

Janet was diagnosed in January 1993 with a glioblastoma, a fast-growing malignancy that attacks the brain and spinal column. Janet's physicians said that she probably had less than a year to live. Nevertheless, Janet endured a standard treatment: first, surgery, then six weeks of radiation therapy. At the end of the six-week period, the tumor was actually larger than it had been before the surgery. Her doctors next suggested radiosurgery (a noninvasive method of destroying tissue within the skull by precisely directing a beam of ionizing radiation), but the family's radiation oncologist said that the tumor had grown too large for that approach. Janet returned to her primary oncologist, who suggested an experimental chemotherapy as the only possible treatment.

Meanwhile, Al had been collecting literature on glioblastomas. He first used the commercial online service CompuServe to search MEDLINE, a huge medical database, and later, with the help of a friend at the National Library of Medicine, compiled his own collection of approximately 1400 MEDLINE references.

Studying the references and using physician contacts on the CompuServe Cancer Forum, Al discovered that the chemotherapy being proposed for Janet had a near-zero probability of saving her life. When he asked why it was being prescribed, he says that the physicians in charge of her treatment told him: "You're basically talking about gaining a few weeks here. *There's nothing else.*"

Instead of accepting this "nothing else" verdict as final, Al, after consultation with family members, used the literature and his online contacts to put together a list of possible treatments. He came up with a list of *over one hundred* possible treatments from around the world. One was an experimental type of radiosurgery, which could be used on tumors too large for standard methods. The family decided to try it. There seemed little to lose. By that time, Janet was disoriented and had difficulty walking, and standard approaches held out almost no hope for her.

The new technique, called fractionated stereotactic radiosurgery, involves attacking the tumor a section at a time with focused radiation. Within weeks of the treatment's completion, Janet's tumor disappeared off the scans. She felt almost well and walked normally again. But the new technique had bought her time, not a cure.

The tumor started growing again, this time in a form too diffuse for more radiosurgery. Al again went through his journal articles and discovered one whose title — something about a chemotherapy's success "in a minority of patients" — almost caused him to overlook it. It turned out that "minority" meant between 30 and 40 percent — a far better rate than the under 5 percent of patients with similarly advanced glioblastomas who had been helped by other chemotherapies.

There was still a problem: the drug in question, tamoxifen, had been used almost exclusively for breast cancer. None of Janet's physicians had ever heard of its use in treating brain tumors. Finally, one agreed to read the article that Al had located and, after talking by phone with the California physician who had written it, authorized the therapy.

Janet's tumor soon stabilized and, after six months, started shrinking. That was over a year ago. That's not long enough to count as a definite "cure," but her ability to walk, talk, and take care of her four children is back to normal. Her only adverse side effect is a partial loss of peripheral vision, due to one of her surgeries.

Al sums up his conclusions succinctly:

"The most important thing is to check out the standard treatments and how well they work. If they work out acceptably, go with them until they stop working. If they don't have a good record, try experimental treatments early. A lot of people wait until too late."

Al Musella's experience shows that a sufficiently determined and well-organized search for information can pay huge dividends even in a life-threatening situation when time is of the essence. He adds that his particular search could not have been conducted in the time available without computers. It was vital that he locate not only recent literature but *the very latest* literature, and finding print references in even an unusually well-stocked library would have been too time-consuming. By using technology effectively, he, a foot doctor, often discovered that he had read articles that brain tumor specialists had not yet found time to read. Databases and online groups complement each other, he says. The information in databases like MEDLINE provides the basic information published in journal articles that physicians respect. The contacts you can make in online groups will help you interpret that information and suggest leads for further research.

WHAT THEY DID, YOU CAN DO

These five stories involve different people, different illnesses, and different aspects of the challenges and rewards that come with becoming an active patient. What they have in common is that all of the people involved made a commitment for themselves or for someone they loved. They refused to settle for second-best treatment. For several of them, that decision was a matter of life or death, for there's every reason to believe that second-best would have been fatal.

You have no guarantee that a comparable effort on your part will lead to the discovery of what the tabloids call a "miracle cure." Nor did these people have any such guarantee. In some instances, they still do not. But they immeasurably improved their chances for a cure by locating the *best* options modern medicine has to offer, and that best is extraordinarily good.

As it happens, all of these individuals experienced difficulties in communicating with at least one physician, but all of them got past that hurdle to take advantage of the skills other physicians could provide. The kind of doctor-patient partnerships they ultimately achieved would not have been possible if they themselves had not shown their own respect for learning and intellectual rigor that characterizes the best physicians.

You may think that you lack some of their training or their resources. Be that as it may, you have other resources. If you feel inadequate, so did they. As these extraordinary people describe their experiences, they often mention a turning point, a moment of almost frightening clarity, when they first realized that they were going to have to take control of crucial treatment decisions. Nothing in their previous ideas about what it means to be a "patient" had prepared them for that. Yet they resolved that somehow they would find out whatever they needed to know. Then, sometimes within a few weeks, sometimes over several years, they did just that.

What they did, you can do.

3.

Medical Stalemates, Moral Victories

NOT EVERY PATIENT who takes an active role in fighting his or her own illness discovers a "miracle" treatment leading to a cure or complete remission. That does happen. It happened for most of the individuals whose stories are told in the preceding chapter. It can happen for you. But no one can guarantee that. Yet this inevitable element of uncertainty in no way reduces the importance of your becoming an active patient.

Often, especially for the most serious illnesses, active patients attain a different kind of victory than any of them would wish as a first choice, but no less miraculous for all that. By refusing to withdraw and give up, many people find hope and courage for themselves and satisfaction in being able to help others.

There's evidence that a positive, optimistic attitude in the face of adversity also produces physiological benefits. That possibility will be considered briefly toward the end of this chapter, but it's neither a certainty nor the main point. The main point is that, although you have no guarantee that becoming an active patient will enable you to discover a medical breakthrough, the decision to do so both increases your chances of finding such a treatment and may in itself restore dignity, hope, and a sense of participation and control over the vital decisions influencing the quality of your life.

"SOMEBODY'S GOING TO DISCOVER SOMETHING . . ."

"I think that most people," says Ronald J. Surface, who was diagnosed in 1988 with Parkinson's disease, "when they are told they have a chronic, debilitating condition, go through a series of emotional states — first denial, then depression, then acceptance. If the diagnosis comes early in the course of the disease, there is a natural tendency to think there must be some mistake. It was that feeling which first caused me to start reading everything I could get my hands on about Parkinson's disease."

Ronald's feeling was understandable. Although Parkinson's disease, a disease of the nervous system, affects about one percent of the population over age 65, Ron began to experience its first symptoms around age 40. Yet the diagnosis was no mistake. Ron acknowledges a period of profound depression, not only from the medication he had begun to take but from the grim long-term prognosis presented in the medical literature. (Suicide, he notes, is a common cause of death for Parkinson's disease patients.)

Ron had divided his career between teaching and service as an Army National Guard officer on active duty. His diagnosis came from doctors at a U.S. Army hospital, and most of his treatments have been by Army physicians. Here is Ron's own crisp summary of his experience:

"Military doctors are usually good, but they seldom have enough time to spend on individual patients, and military patients don't often get to see the same doctor on follow-up visits. In addition, treatment in military hospitals tends to be somewhat conservative. I soon determined that if I were going to learn anything, I would have to do it myself. I began searching on MEDLINE and soon discovered an experimental drug which offered the hope of slowing the progress of the disease. I was able to convince my attending physician to try it, and I am happy to report it is reasonably successful. The Army has since placed me on disability retirement, and I have continued to search the literature. I have discovered several research programs exploring new treatment protocols for Parkinson's, and I am currently exploring the possibility of becoming a participant in one of them."

Physicians who are wary of encouraging patients to read technical literature on their illnesses sometimes quote Alexander Pope's famous line, "A little learning is a dangerous thing." Ron agrees, but the moral he draws is not that you shouldn't start reading; rather, you should keep at it. He did. "Finally," he writes in a letter to the authors, "as I became aware of some of the promising research being done and the encouraging results of some of the research, I was able to accept my condition."

Ron continues to monitor medical literature as fast as it appears in print — sometimes faster, since some databases contain leads to unpublished research in progress. Calling computers "the ultimate form of handicap access," he does information searches both for himself and for others. Many of his clients are physicians who respect his skill at finding information.

Ron's strategy is to keep himself as healthy as possible while medical science advances and, of course, to make sure that he knows about advances as they occur. It's not only a rational strategy in terms of his physical health; following it has helped to keep him mentally healthy.

"I am certainly glad," he concludes, "I didn't accept the conventional wisdom that Parkinson's disease is relentlessly progressive and that there is nothing we can do about it. I am constantly asking my doctor, 'Have you read about . . . ?' If he hasn't read the material in question, I go to the medical library and get a copy for him. He may not have time to find all the relevant articles, but I have a lot of time. There would not be much to look forward to if I did not believe that continued research can make a difference. Somebody's going to discover something, and I want to be in line for it."

LEARNING TO COPE WITHOUT A MEDICAL MIRACLE

Bonnie Hatfield, who lives in Half Moon Bay, California, also suffers from a progressive disease for which there is, at present, no "magic bullet." For a time she suffered from passive acceptance of her symptoms as well, letting family and friends convince her that her problems were normal for her age. She's not only moved beyond that attitude for herself; she's actively engaged in helping fellow patients around the world to cope with their symptoms and to monitor ongoing medical research.

In 1983 Bonnie, then in her early forties and a single mother with teenage children, began feeling "monumental" fatigue. After a week's work, she was so tired that she'd have to spend weekends in bed. Tendinitis brought pain to her shoulders. She began dropping things.

"I had to plan my life very meticulously," she says, "so that I could get through the day. Carrying groceries into the house was an ordeal. I would sometimes fall down. Or I'd get stuck on a stairway. I'd get halfway up and my legs would just quit."

When she was eleven years old, Bonnie had been stricken with polio, only a few years before the introduction of the Salk vaccine began to eradicate the disease in the United States. It never occurred to her that there might be a connection between her present symptoms and a viral disease that had attacked her over thirty years earlier and from which she thought she had made a complete recovery.

No one encouraged her to ask questions or even to see a doctor. Friends convinced her that her fatigue was normal. She was, they pointed out, working hard (first as the financial manager of a computer software firm, later in her own consulting business), rearing adolescent children, keeping up a household, and going through menopause. Her teenagers, preoccupied with their own lives, told her, "Mom, it's just old age."

In 1988 she moved to the San Francisco area, where one friend took her seriously. This woman, after a search through a popular medical library, mailed her photocopies of three articles on a disease called postpoliomyelitis syndrome, usually shortened to postpolio syndrome (PPS). The friend added a note: "It sounds like you have this."

"I cried when I read them," Bonnie says. "Everything in them pertained to me."

Belatedly, Bonnie consulted a physician, who agreed that she had PPS, a recurrence of neuromuscular symptoms in acute polio victims, often after many years have elapsed. The connection is not always obvious because the disease does not necessarily strike only those limbs once affected by polio.

Bonnie immediately began her own search of the medical literature, first at the library her friend had consulted, later at the Lane Medical Library at Stanford University. MEDLINE was available only to Stanford students and faculty, so she painstakingly looked up references at the end of those articles she had and found new ones by reading the tables of contents of new medical journals on the library's shelves. Slowly, she compiled an extensive collection of articles on PPS. She recalls how she'd spend a half day at the library and then return home to spend the rest of the day in bed in complete exhaustion.

She often does that still.

In physical terms, Bonnie's story does not yet have a happy ending. No treatment is known for reversing the damage done by PPS, and few treatments offer much relief. She sometimes still feels fatigue so severe that it brings on nausea. Driving a car is difficult, and carrying in groceries remains an ordeal. Even prolonged speech is an effort, because her diaphragm muscles tire.

She says that she could have taken better care of herself if she'd started to ask questions sooner but regards none of her recent research effort as wasted. It's had one unexpected and positive side effect: she's become the center of an international correspondence group. Some years back, when Bonnie had located approximately twenty articles on postpolio syndrome, she decided she ought to share them. With the encouragement of friends, she began mailing photocopies of a bibliography to anyone who requested it. That bibliography has grown to forty pages and now contains about five hundred articles. She still sends it out for a modest handling charge, often with photocopies of articles.

As a result, Bonnie gets letters from around the world. Her correspondents offer encouragement and suggestions on how to cope with fatigue problems — sometimes on ordinary matters like how to schedule rest periods throughout the day. They tell Bonnie that she was fortunate in one respect: that the physician she consulted gave her a prompt and accurate diagnosis — possibly because she came prepared with literature. Many say that their physicians, unfamiliar with PPS, often dismissed symptoms with "It's all in your head" or "It's normal for your age," much as Bonnie's own teenagers once did. Her accomplishments, achieved despite severe physical problems, show that it's never too late to benefit from becoming an active patient.

Like Ron Surface, Bonnie monitors current medical developments closely. So far, her only tangible benefits are improved coping skills and a recognition on the part of family and friends that her symptoms have a real physiological basis. She takes even more satisfaction from "being part of the give-and-take for this PPS community all over the world." Finally, like Ron, she remains hopeful. As a result of her efforts, she knows that if a medical breakthrough on postpolio syndrome occurs anywhere in the world, she'll be one of the first people to hear about it.

CHRONICALLY FATIGUED BUT AN ONLINE ACTIVIST

Valerie Ostroth, who lives in Blacksburg, Virginia, has physical problems resembling Bonnie Hatfield's. Her response has been similar, except that she's been able to take full advantage of computers for both research and breaking through potential isolation. She remembers exactly when her first symptoms hit her — June 4, 1991, at 4 P.M.

"I was mowing the church lawn with a push mower," she writes in a letter recalling the experience, "and just collapsed. It was like a sudden energy drain."

She was rushed to her doctor, and she and he both suspected that she might have contracted Rocky Mountain spotted fever from a tick bite. Because there seemed no time for extensive tests, she was put immediately on antibiotics. She remained bedridden for a week with "horrible flu-like symptoms" that included nausea, dizziness, a sore throat, swollen glands, and alternating fever and chills.

Valerie teaches English at Virginia Polytechnic Institute and State University, located in Blacksburg, and is comfortable using a computer. As soon as possible, working from her office, she began using a university machine to search some of the online databases (databases searchable over telephone lines) described in later chapters. She checked out information on Rocky Mountain spotted fever and Lyme disease.

She tried going back to work at the beginning of the fall semester but developed new symptoms on top of the fatigue, fever, and chills.

"I was weak," she writes. "My digestive system was at war with me, my mind was 'losing it,' and I had trouble talking. I also began to black out, forget my way home, and collapse every day, midday, and early evening until the next day. By October, it was clear I was unable to continue teaching."

She went on extended sick leave but borrowed a computer from the university to finish some projects at home. She also used it to continue searching databases. Valerie already had, and still retains, a wonderful working relationship with her primary care physician, who had been her doctor for thirteen years. He was, she says, "very responsive and also not threatened by my quest for as much information as possible through the databases. Many friends have since told me that their docs have not been as comfortable with patients' knowledge searching."

In September, her doctor had mentioned that he was beginning to suspect her problem was not Rocky Mountain spotted fever, but chronic fatigue and immune dysfunction syndrome (CFIDS) (often shortened to chronic fatigue syndrome, or CFS), a condition of uncertain cause characterized by disabling fatigue after a viral-like illness.

"He first suspected," says Valerie, "following an Epstein-Barr titer test which was way above normal, but not necessarily indicative of CFIDS. He said the Center for Disease Control (CDC) definition requires a minimum of six months of illness before the official diagnosis.

"I had been a high-energy person," she explains, "volunteering for lots of fun things, teaching a full load, mothering, gardening, etc. And now I was a shadow of my former self. . . . The symptoms by now included weakness in my extremities, trouble with hand coordination (I couldn't hold eating utensils at all — people probably thought I was drunk), more memory/cognition problems, increased sensitivity to food allergies, sleep disturbances, weight gain, sensitivity to light, and a general fog over my brain."

She recalls all this with some precision because she kept a record of it. Later, she discovered in online databases that all of these symptoms were part of the official CFIDS definition. Six months passed, and at the beginning of 1992, "I was official."

Soon after that, she had to return the university computer, but her parents and husband, seeing how much it had meant to her, got together to buy a computer for her use at home. Searching databases, she came across repeated references to an internationally recognized specialist in CFIDS, Dr. Paul Cheney, who, as luck would have it, had recently moved from Nevada to nearby North Carolina. With the "blessings and good wishes" of her family physician, she consulted Dr. Cheney.

After giving her six days of tests, Dr. Cheney talked with her "nonstop for four hours." They talked about what she'd learned in her searches. "Without that background and the immersion into the databases," she says, "I would've been clueless about what he was telling me."

She now takes an extensive range of medications and vitamins. Although her sleep has improved, most of her symptoms remain. But she takes encouragement from knowing that the medical literature indicates that most CFIDS patients recover in about five years; she's at the three-year point. "Perhaps," she concludes, "every day is a day toward recovery! That's what I have to believe, but if not, I am learning to adapt and live as fully as I can under the circumstances."

Because of the stress that CFIDS brings to families, Valerie's family has been seeing a family therapist together. The therapist has asked Valerie to help her write a book on the effects of chronic illness on family and friends. "She is fascinated," Valerie writes, "with the info I get from the computer searches. . . . We may get her online soon!"

Valerie herself is online a lot. Although she emphasizes that her grasp of searching electronically is limited, she's learned how to communicate with an online discussion group for CFS/CFIDS patients, family members, and physicians, in which she is an active participant.

36 ■ INFOMEDICINE

"When I'm not able to put words into sentences because part of my illness is like a brain injury that affects my ability to communicate verbally," Valerie says, "I can sit down at the terminal, and the computer doesn't care how fast or how slow I type something out. A lot of people have acknowledged that's how they use it, too. There might be a time when they can't talk on the phone or meet face-to-face, and the computer is there when they need it."

Today she's in almost daily contact with people around the world who share her problems. She acquires early insights on the benefits, and risks, of drugs and treatment therapies not yet approved for CFS/CFIDS use in the United States.

"It was very helpful," she says, "to get a worldwide perspective on this illness, and it was also very reassuring to know that I wasn't alone, because my social contact has dropped significantly since I became ill. We PWCs [persons with CFS/CFIDS] are often so alienated or alone that the human contact is vital for the survival of our minds."

That, perhaps, is the main point of her story. She has reason to believe that her symptoms will abate and perhaps vanish in time. Meanwhile, she's not letting them cut her off from the world. The very process of becoming an active patient has already guaranteed that.

THE MIND-BODY CONNECTION

Ron Surface, Bonnie Hatfield, and Valerie Ostroth, despite the severity of their disorders, have gained some physical benefits from their determined searches for treatments better than those first offered them. They have located physicians who will work closely with them or medications that alleviate some symptoms. They continue to look for even more promising treatments. The most striking aspect of their stories is the emotional strength they have derived from becoming active participants in their own medical care.

Meanwhile, an increasing body of evidence suggests that emotional strength becomes part of the equation for physical survival or improvement during illness. There are a number of reasons for this, but the most obvious is simply that it's far better to feel in control than to feel the stress associated with being dependent and powerless. It is clear that there is link between mind and body, a biochemical association between the brain and the other organs. An obvious example of this is the prickly "adrenaline surge" you feel when sudden danger looms, such as a car swerving into your path.

Can stress hasten the progress of disease, and can the absence of stress inhibit that progress? Evidence suggests that the answer to both questions is "yes," although nobody knows to what degree this is so. Within a new discipline called psychoneuroimmunology — the study of the interaction between the nervous, endocrine, and immune systems — scientists have recently begun to explore that connection.

In a laboratory experiment performed in the 1980s, a group of mice were injected with tumor cells and then exposed to stress (in the form of electric shock) from which they could escape with relative ease. A second group was also subjected to shock but not provided with the means of escaping it. At the end of the experiment, the mice were examined for the extent of tumor growth. Those who experienced escapable stress showed a delayed increase in tumor development, while the group unable to escape shock did not. The experiment suggests that the key factor in enhanced tumor development was not stress itself but the *inability to control it*.

Results published in 1992 of an experiment on the effect of stress upon the immune system proved that in a group of medical students tested, stress was clearly related to the subjects' ability to generate antibody response to a vaccine. Moreover, another factor — social support — also played a key role. Students who scored higher on a scale measuring such factors as their sense of belonging and self-esteem showed stronger immune response than students situated lower on the scale.

Even though the full extent of the mind-body relationship is still somewhat of a mystery, the benefits of being well informed about your medical condition are clear. For example, cancer surgeon Dr. Bernie Siegel — author of *Love, Medicine, and Miracles* — has classified patients into three types: passive, concerned consumers, and active. The first group he describes as "resigned," the second as "obedient" and completely focused on getting approval from their doctors. But those in the last group, he says, become intensely involved in learning and reading everything they can about their condition. They query their physicians for clarification in order to work with them, and they refuse to give up control of their own situation.

The physical course of illness among the three groups, according to Siegel's experience and other health studies, varies dramatically. The first group has the worst outcomes; the second, average; and the last — those who have been in control by becoming involved in treatment decision-making — the best.

Whatever scientists may yet discover about the nature of mind-body links, for people like Surface, Hatfield, and Ostroth, the word "victim" already seems inappropriate. What they lack in certainty of cure they make up in courage and refusal to withdraw into themselves. Although they have yet to overcome their physical disorders, they have already prevailed against their disorders' soul-crushing effects. And their methodical searches for treatment options played a central role in those moral and psychological victories, enabling them to help many other people even while improving the odds for themselves.

PART II

YOU CAN DO

EFFECTIVE RESEARCH

Finding the best treatment may be easier than you think. First of all, you'll aim for an active partnership with your physician, making clear that you're prepared to do your part in working toward that goal. Although the electronic resources discussed later are growing in importance, there is a wealth of information available in medical libraries and from hundreds of health-related organizations. Even if you have no medical training, you can learn to use all of these resources effectively.

4.

Doctor-Patient Relationships

THE RELATIONSHIP YOU forge with your physician will play a key role in the outcome of your pursuit for the most effective treatment. It is clearly one of the most productive alliances you can have.

Good doctors have always recognized this. Sixty years ago, Dr. Francis Peabody, professor of medicine at Harvard Medical School, stood before his students and described what he called the "crux of the whole situation" of caring for patients: "The significance of the intimate personal relationship between physician and patient cannot be too strongly emphasized . . . both diagnosis and treatment are directly dependent on it."

Dr. Peabody was speaking long before specialization and high-technology medicine had begun to overshadow the private, one-on-one aspect of the doctor-patient relationship, but his message is equally pertinent today.

"Patients," says Thomas Delbanco, M.D., in a key study on the doctor-patient relationship published in *Annals of Internal Medicine* (March 1992), " . . . are concerned about issues of clinical significance that have nothing to do with what we think of as the doctor's 'image.' They want to be able to trust the competence and efficiency of their caregivers."

Delbanco continues with a quote from a patient interviewed for the study: "I feel very strongly that the patient has to participate. . . . This is not a theoretical thing. I have learned that I have to be as involved in my care as the doctors."

Unfortunately, however, physicians often have no way of knowing how much patients want to learn about their medical condition. If patients *don't* ask questions, it's easy for a doctor to assume that the patient is apathetic or simply wants to be told how to proceed with the treatment. "The important thing is for patients to express their interest," says Brenda A., a young pediatrician in group practice. "If they don't do that, I respond as a human and think they don't want as much information, and maybe I don't give them as much as I would with someone who is really showing interest."

It's important, therefore, to explain to the doctor that you're probably not the average patient and want to be an active participant in your treatment decisions. Let the doctor know that if you ask a lot of questions it is not to challenge, but rather to educate yourself. Say that you are eager to get detailed information during the visit and plan to continue learning as much as possible about your condition on your own. Explain that you know your doctor's time is valuable and that you will make every effort to prepare yourself prior to office visits to use that time as effectively as possible.

HEALTH HISTORY-TAKING

Your first opportunity for real communication with your physician is likely to be when he "takes your history" — that is, learns something about you, the reason for your visit, and your symptoms. The health history-taking procedure may look simple and straightforward, but in fact it requires great skill. What appears to be an apparently seamless succession of questions is really a carefully constructed scrutiny of explicit, individual aspects of your health history and present physical condition. Proper diagnosis often rests upon your physician's ability to synthesize and correctly interpret the information gathered during this procedure.

The interview, consequently, should take place in an atmosphere that includes a sense of privacy in surroundings, an absence of interruptions, direct eye contact (you and your doctor at the same level), and an attentive, unhurried atmosphere.

Initial impressions often set the tone of the relationship. It is at this time that your physician will first judge your ability and desire to communicate. The best physicians use this opportunity to convey the impression that they see their patients as individuals, not as abstract clinical cases.

It is also your opportunity to observe your doctor and ascertain her level of concern and commitment.

"The first question I ask," says the pediatrician quoted earlier, "is always something like, 'What's the problem? What's concerning you?' This lets my patients know that *their* concerns are the most important thing to me, and it gets our meeting on a proper footing."

All patient histories include certain elements:

- *identifying data* — age, sex, place of birth, occupation, and so forth.
- *reason for visit* — checkup or specific complaint.
- *description of symptoms* — a detailed account of the primary reason the patient is seeking care (chest pain, sore throat, and so forth), including, for example, onset of the problem, circumstances in which it developed, quality and timing ("Is the pain sharp or dull?" "How often?"), description of increase or decrease in symptoms (walking up the stairs, feeling stressed), and secondary symptoms (general fatigue, fever, and so forth).

As much as possible, your doctor should let you recount your story without interruption. This allows your narrative — with all the important details that may be critical to your doctor's accurate diagnosis — to unfold naturally and spontaneously.

This rarely happens without some interruption and prompting, however, and the best doctors will perform that function skillfully — for example, "Where did it hurt when you said you 'woke up in pain'?" or, to break a silence, your doctor might encourage you to continue by saying, "I'm listening" or "Please go on."

Calling for an elaboration is also an important skill. To illustrate, some symptoms of heart disease can also be symptoms of other problems. If a patient simply says he is short of breath, it rests with the doctor to narrow down the possibilities. "I might ask a patient how that problem affects his usual activity — what it prevents him from doing," notes Dr. Urs Leuenberger, a cardiologist who teaches and practices at a university hospital.

A careful doctor will not lead you but might ask, "What color was the phlegm you coughed up?" rather than "Was the phlegm you coughed up red?" Thoroughness is another key component of a well-executed history-taking. A conscientious doctor will give you an additional chance to mention something you may have forgotten or were possibly reluctant at first to talk about. Dr. Robert Dye, an internist in private practice for thirty years, remarks: "I usually say, 'Have we covered everything we should have covered? Have we left out anything?' "

After your present illness is discussed, your doctor then should proceed to take your past history (previous illnesses, injuries, operations) and current health status (allergies; immunizations; results of any previous tests or screenings; exercise, sleep, and diet; current medications; and so forth). Also included would be your family history (ages and present health or cause of death; incidence of specific diseases, such as diabetes, high blood pressure, alcoholism, and so forth, to reveal possible risk factors).

The final part of a good health-history interview consists of specific questions — called the "review of systems" — about different anatomical regions, such as eye, ear, gastrointestinal, and so forth. Its purpose is to draw out information you might not initially have provided.

During the history-taking, make the effort to judge the style and thoroughness of your physician. He may be a model of efficiency and caring, and all you have to do is to respond. But be alert. If you realize that the history-taking is about to move beyond an area where you have more to add, speak up; you may be distracted and later forget something you need to say.

PHYSICAL EXAMINATION

The physical examination verifies the presence or absence of medical conditions inferred from the history interview, and plays the final critical role in obtaining an appropriate diagnosis.

A considerate doctor will remember during the examination to tell you exactly what he is doing, and alert you to possible discomfort. He should reassure you that things are going smoothly or, if he discovers something, avoid alarming you. ("There's a little patch here I'll go back and check, and we'll talk about it then"). All the while the physician notes your body signs and conditions in order to write them into the record immediately after the examination. (Some physicians dictate notes to a nurse or assistant as they go along.)

If this is your first visit for a specific medical problem, your doctor may wish to check several major body systems, such as pulmonary, cardiovascular, musculoskeletal, endocrine, gastrointestinal, hepatic, neurologic, or reproductive. Diseases of these various body systems often manifest themselves with similar symptoms. A proper differential diagnosis requires that your doctor be thorough and attentive to their complex interrelationships. (A differential diagnosis determines which of two or more diseases with similar symptoms is the one from which you may be suffering.)

AN EXAMPLE OF A DOCTOR WHO COMMUNICATED WELL

What do we want from doctors? The experience of Walter, who sought medical help for a pressing problem from internist Ken Bailey, offers a strong example of a near-ideal doctor-patient relationship.

"Although I'm only twenty-nine," says Walter, "I believed I had some of the danger signs of colon cancer — bleeding and a recent change in bowel habits. Also, my grandfather and father had both died of colon cancer, and I knew that sometimes it tends to run in families."

At the suggestion of a colleague, Walter called Dr. Ken Bailey, an internist at a teaching hospital. He explained his concern to the receptionist and briefly outlined his symptoms, then asked for an appointment.

"The receptionist said he didn't have any openings for six weeks," he recalls, "and all I could think of was that early detection is important in curing colon cancer. So I asked her if she'd specifically mention my concerns to the doctor, as well as my symptoms, and find out if he thought it could wait six weeks."

The receptionist called Walter back. Although there was nothing to be alarmed about, based on his symptoms, she said, the doctor wanted to see him soon. The receptionist gave Walter an appointment for the following week and instruction in preparing for examination.

"The first time I saw the doctor was when he walked into the examining room. He gave me a firm handshake, sat down opposite me, and said, 'Now, tell me the story.' He let me talk for about five minutes, taking some notes. I described my symptoms, and once in a while he'd ask a question — about my diet, or whether I ever felt any pain in my abdomen, for instance."

Walter says that Dr. Bailey never seemed bored or in a hurry, took his history carefully, and gave him a head-to-toe physical, explaining what he was doing as he went along. At the end of the physical, Dr. Bailey told Walter that he seemed healthy. He added, however, that in order to rule out the possibility that Walter might have a potentially cancerous polyp in his colon, he would like to do a sigmoidoscopy there in the office. The procedure, Dr. Bailey explained, involves examining the lower bowel with a flexible fiber-optic probe.

"He told me," Walter says, "the primary danger of the procedure (perforation) and that it was rare. 'In my career, I've done twenty-five hundred of these and have never perforated,' he told me. 'And my patients always tell me that it wasn't bad at all. As we go along, I'll let you know when there are a couple of painful turns, and if you say the word, I'll back off and let you take a breather.'

"Then Dr. Bailey asked me if I had any remaining questions. After I asked a few, which he answered carefully, I signed a 'consent' form that stated that I agreed to undergo the procedure and that I understood its risks."

The examination proceeded smoothly. Walter felt "surprisingly relaxed" and never felt it necessary to ask for the promised "breather." "I trusted Dr. Bailey," he says, "because of the way he had presented everything to me."

The outcome for Walter was a happy one. The bleeding, he learned, was caused by small fissures — not polyps — and the other changes were within a normal range that could be modified by diet.

Walter's story illustrates an almost perfect instance of good doctor-patient communication. Not only was the doctor conscientious, attentive, and supportive, but the patient was informed and given some degree of control over what could have been an uncomfortable procedure.

HOW POOR COMMUNICATION MAY FORCE A CHANGE OF DOCTORS

Laurel Simmons, already introduced in an earlier chapter, was twenty-four when some problems in recovering from wisdom-tooth extraction caused her to be referred for blood testing and then to an oncologist, Dr. M., for further examination. He diagnosed CML (chronic myelogenous leukemia).

"Dr. M. was a well-known specialist in the Boston area," Laurel says,

> and connected with one of its most prestigious hospitals. The clinic where I saw him was very busy. One afternoon, a nurse informed me that there were nineteen patients waiting for him.
>
> I made it clear to him from the beginning that I wanted to know as much as I could concerning my disease. But he was very pressed for time. He acted as though my questions were an imposition to him. There were always nurses coming in. He was always answering the phone and having conversa-

tions with other patients. All of this made me feel that it was not acceptable for me to pursue a question with him.

Right after he gave me the diagnosis, he said, "What we're going to do now is get you a bone marrow transplant." And that was that. There was no discussion. I was young and had never been seriously ill, so I didn't have an idea of what to expect when a doctor talked to me.

As soon as she was diagnosed and told she needed a bone marrow transplant (BMT), a group of Laurel's friends at the Massachusetts Institute of Technology, where she worked, formed a support group for her and began gathering medical information about BMTs. One of them mentioned some literature that suggested the procedure might cause sterility.

"At my next visit, I asked Dr. M. what my post-BMT fertility would be and whether or not I should harvest my eggs beforehand. He said, 'Don't worry about it. Fifteen percent of women can have babies after BMT, and since you're young and healthy, you'll probably be one of them.' "

Laurel told her friends. They soon learned that at that time (1987), the research showed that girls who hadn't begun to menstruate when they received a BMT went on to have children years later. "But there was no instance," she continues, "of any woman ever having had a baby if she had her BMT after puberty. When Dr. M. told me about that fifteen percent, he must have included the children, and he just said it as a way of deflecting my question. If he could do that, how was he answering any other questions I had about my treatment? I lost faith in him completely and decided to find another oncologist."

Laurel found a new doctor, also a busy specialist at one of Boston's great teaching hospitals, who confirmed her first oncologist's recommendations on the bone marrow transplant. But her thoughts about harvesting eggs had now been pushed out of her mind. She was weary of the stress of preparing for a procedure that at that time was still very risky. She had found a donor (one of her brothers) and was eager to put the ordeal of the BMT behind her. By then her emotions had been refocused, and the time in which to make a momentous decision had been lost.

If you've done your share in opening communications, as Laurel did, but your doctor makes you feel nervous or uneasy and tends to give abrupt, unsatisfactory, or cursory answers, it will be difficult to become an active participant in your medical care. Being able to research material related to your condition on your own is important, but it is of little help if you're working with a doctor whose advice you don't completely trust. If you find yourself in this circumstance, seriously consider finding another physician.

GOOD COMMUNICATION IS A TWO-WAY STREET

Our final example illustrates a situation where both physician and patient may have been partially responsible for a tragic breakdown in communication.

For two months, Robert Kephart had been plagued by severe abdominal pain. His internist had run tests for abnormalities in his gastrointestinal tract, but the results were negative. Nevertheless, the internist prescribed a medication to block gastric acid output, thinking the problem was related to an ulcerative type of condition that the tests hadn't identified. But Robert's condition didn't improve. Each time he returned home from a visit to the doctor, his wife, Mary, asked: "Did you tell him how sick you're feeling?" Robert always answered that he had.

Still, the doctor made no new suggestions about what was causing the pain, and Robert's condition worsened. "He used to roll up in a ball when he came home from work," recalls Mary, "and one day he spent four hours almost in tears.

"Finally," she says, "I went with him to his doctor's appointment. Nothing much happened. The doctor didn't appear focused on what seemed a terrible problem for my husband. He gave us about 2 percent of his attention. At last, I spoke up and described my husband's pain — telling him how Robert rolled up into a ball and how sometimes he could hardly keep from crying. Finally, the doctor looked at me and said, 'I had no idea it was like that.' "

Mary pressed her husband's physician for further tests. The doctor immediately made an appointment with a specialist to test for pancreas involvement. The results revealed that Robert was suffering from pancreatic cancer, and an exploratory operation showed his case to be too far advanced for surgery.

The doctor didn't know that Robert's pain was severe enough to make him curl himself into a ball or come close to tears with anguish. Robert, a retired military officer, may have been reluctant to suggest any sign of weakness. But by failing to be specific about his symptoms, he very likely conveyed that he was not as sick as he actually felt. Nevertheless, as Mary points out, his doctor had a responsibility to elicit more information when her husband clearly wasn't responding to what is usually a very effective treatment for ulcerative conditions.

As Robert's experience shows, it's a mistake to assume or hope that doctors will draw out all the necessary information every time they take a history. The lesson to be learned carries no less weight because Robert's cancer was undoubtedly too far advanced for it to have affected his prognosis (although clearly a much more aggressive approach could have been taken to relieve his day-to-day pain). Under any circumstances, it cannot be stressed too strongly that the part you play in communicating everything you can about your condition is of immense significance.

Always make a full disclosure of all your symptoms and any other medically related problems that you may have. Noel Ballentine, M.D., an internist who teaches and practices at an academic medical center, characterizes the issue this way:

> The doctor-patient relationship is the core of good medicine, to be sure. On the part of the patient, there must be honesty and full disclosure. To help, physicians must know exactly where the patient is coming from. Over 50 percent of the time patients do not tell doctors everything they know about their symptoms. The reasons include fear of a dreaded diagnosis, embarrassment, preset notions about which symptoms are important, and so forth. I cannot help an alcoholic who will not tell me he has a problem.

Dr. Ballentine's view, held by most physicians, is one of being committed to helping all patients — even those who don't offer full cooperation. But he emphasizes that a doctor's efforts at providing the best medical care are impeded by a patient who is not forthright.

TECHNIQUES FOR BETTER DOCTOR-PATIENT RELATIONSHIPS

Different individuals, doctors and patients alike, have different communication styles and communication skills. Fortunately, a good doctor-patient relationship is not totally dependent on personalities or habitual ways of speaking. Your physician may not be as empathic and warm as Walter's internist (nor, in all probability, will he be as brusque and cold as Laurel's first oncologist), but you can do several things to improve the chances of a sound, long-term relationship.

The Time Factor

Physicians in general feel pressured by the clock. They may have a large practice, be members of a group plan with economic incentives that require their seeing large numbers of patients, have to make extensive hospital rounds, or — as in academic medicine — carry a full teaching load. The one place where they can relieve that pressure is in the length of time spent with patients during office hours. And they often do. While this may not seem fair, it is also a fact of life. In the long run, your recognition that time with the doctor is limited will help by forcing you to become a more effective patient and make the most of your office visits.

Preparing for Your Office Visit

When you go to the doctor's office, for example, plan to take a notepad listing your symptoms and questions. List the symptoms and questions in separate sections. Leave plenty of space between the questions for answers, and date all entries.

Some points to remember:

• The first notebook entry for your visit should provide details of the primary complaint. When did it start? When does it occur? Are your symptoms getting worse? and so forth.

• Next, include *any* other changes in your health or physical habits. Let the doctor decide what is important and what is not.

• Write down all the prescription medications you are taking, especially whether you *always* take them as prescribed, and — most important — whether you've had any recent dosage changes. If you can't read the labels, bring the containers along with you to the doctor. Also note any over-the-counter drugs you may be taking.

• When you list your questions, start with the ones you consider most important. It's easy to get distracted during an office visit. When you're on your way home from an appointment is not the time to remember that important question you wished to ask.

During the Office Visit

If someone other than your doctor — such as a nurse or resident — takes your preliminary history, use your notes. Remember to be as thorough and factually accurate with nurses and residents as you plan to be with your doctor. The information they record is usually incorporated as part of your permanent patient record, and busy physicians often rely on it to help pave the way for a productive visit.

When you do see your physician:

• Immediately explain what is bothering you the most. Don't confuse the issue and waste time by discussing, for example, your arthritis if you are there because your main symptom is a sharp pain in the abdomen.

• After explaining your symptoms and their history, check your notepad and make sure you didn't miss anything.

• Above all, be honest. If you haven't kept up with your blood pressure medication, admit it.

• If you are uncomfortable or apprehensive during the examination, ask the doctor to help you.

• Keep notes of any new questions that arise during the visit.

- Write down the diagnosis — or list of possible diagnoses, if the doctor is not sure. Don't try to rely on your memory.
- If you are diagnosed with an acute disease, be sure to ask when to expect to see an improvement with the prescribed treatment.
- Ask how long you should wait to call if your condition does not clear up.
- If a new drug is prescribed, ask about its side effects and interaction with other medications you are taking.
- If the doctor orders a test, ask about its purpose and accuracy. Also tell the doctor you want a photocopy of the test results when they come in, and that you'd like to receive a written evaluation. Certainly if the results are in any way abnormal, you should hear it from the doctor directly so that you can ask questions immediately.

Taking Someone with You

If you feel this is too much to remember or that you need the support and judgment of someone you trust, consider asking a family member or friend to accompany you to the doctor's office and share that responsibility. Justice Sandra Day O'Connor has said of her experience with cancer: "I discovered I needed other ears than my own, because I was so emotionally involved in this situation that I wasn't sure I was hearing everything. I brought my husband along [to meet with doctors] because I thought he could listen with greater objectivity than I could, and we both tried to take a few notes so we got everything down."

Medical Records

If you have a complicated illness requiring a second opinion or multiple visits to several doctors, you should maintain your own medical file. Kim Brady, who has been treated for twenty years for complications related to a defective heart valve, has devised an effective system:

"I get copies of all my records as I go along and organize them into a three-ring binder, marking it off with index tabs so I can locate specific things quickly. When I go to see a specialist, I take the binder along. Doctors can look at the whole thing or whatever is pertinent to them. Sometimes they don't look at it but simply ask me if I've had a certain test or can recall something about my symptoms. I just tab through the binder and find it right away."

Not all records are as complex as Kim's. But you will find that creating a file, at least for your home records, provides valuable reference information for studying your illness and its various treatment options.

You are always entitled to ask for a copy of your medical records. Bear in mind, however, that you normally can't take the *original* documents out of the doctor's office.

What If Your Symptoms Don't Subside?

In some cases, this may not be your first visit to the doctor for a chief complaint that still persists.

Remember that you know your own body best. If you continue to feel that something is wrong and your symptoms don't subside following treatment, or your physician says that test results are negative and your symptoms will "go away," it's imperative that you persevere in getting an answer or else seek a second opinion. The consequences could be serious if you don't.

Elizabeth, a forty-one-year-old mother of three who lives in the Midwest, complained of irregular bleeding between periods. Although she felt sure there was a problem — she had never experienced such spotting before — the doctor said that the Pap test was normal. But her symptoms did not abate, and although she visited her physician twice again, he wasn't concerned. "You're taking this minimal bleeding too seriously," he told her. "Go home and ignore it."

After a year, Elizabeth decided to seek the help of another doctor, even though her insurance didn't cover the visit. He discovered a grapefruit-sized tumor at the tip of her uterus. After a biopsy and X-rays, Elizabeth received her diagnosis: endometrial carcinoma, with spreading to the lungs.

Elizabeth's condition, adenocarcinoma of the uterus, is not readily detectable with a Pap test. But there are other ways to diagnose it. One method is an endometrial biopsy, a common, relatively noninvasive procedure that can be performed in the doctor's office. Her physician simply did not follow up on Elizabeth's complaint as closely as he should have.

"It's not uncommon to see a missed diagnosis," says Harold B., an obstetrician/gynecologist in private group practice for the past twenty years. "The vast majority of patients who make an appointment because they fear having a serious illness do not actually have one. Maybe physicians, knowing that, tend to ignore the possibility that *this* time there may, indeed, be a serious problem." On that basis, he concludes, the patient would do well to speak up to make the doctor pay attention.

Don't be reluctant to call your physician for another appointment if you have a persistent problem. If you take the advice given earlier, you will have set up parameters for a follow-up phone call during your appointment by asking, "When should I see an improvement? What are the expected side effects of the drug or treatment? How long should I wait before I call?" Contacting your physician in these circumstances is simply following the doctor's orders.

Remember that being an active patient begins with taking responsibility. Ensuring that you obtain an adequate diagnosis is essential to that process.

CHANGING DOCTORS

What if, like Laurel Simmons, you feel that you've done your share in opening communications, and you still don't trust your relationship with your doctor? You know it's time to change; how do you find another doctor? What do you do about your records?

Probably the best way to select a new doctor is to get recommendations from someone you trust, including, if possible, any medical professionals you know. Physician directories, such as those described in the next chapter, as well as online contacts described later may be helpful in identifying specialists.

The chief thing to remember is that it would not be prudent to sever your relationship with one physician, especially your primary care physician, before being accepted by another. You don't want to put yourself in a situation where, in case of emergency, there is no one you can refer to as "your" doctor.

It makes sense, therefore, to begin checking out your options for a transfer as soon as you conclude that it may be necessary. If you are part of a managed-care plan, bear in mind that you will need approval from a plan's administrators to change physicians. This is usually easy where primary care physicians are concerned, but you may find it extremely difficult to be reimbursed for the specialist of your choice. The problems of insurance and managed care are discussed in a later chapter, but clearly you need to know the rules of any plan of which you are a member.

≫≪

Your new physician will assist you in acquiring your medical records. Since medical records are legally the property of the patient, their full release will require a written request from you. In some cases, a physician will honor the request prior to receiving your written permission, in order to expedite the transfer. Note that if you have copies of your records, as suggested earlier in the chapter, you needn't wait for them to be transferred to make your new appointment.

Ask your new doctor to let you see what has been transferred, a request to which he or she normally will not object. The reason for this is that the term "medical records" is in fact somewhat ambiguous. Some physicians maintain records that are only a telegraphic summary of actions taken: for example, "Patient complained of pain in lower abdomen," the names of tests performed and their results, and prescribed medications. Notes gathered during history-taking are often summarized when placed in the record. The point is, of course, that you should never assume that "transfer of records" means that your new doctor will know what you told your old doctor. A physician who communicates poorly with you is likely to communicate equally badly with your new physician.

On the whole, however, changing doctors is not difficult. In fact, the biggest obstacle is most often the patient's reluctance either to hurt the doctor's feelings or simply to make the effort.

Those kinds of considerations clearly aren't appropriate for an active patient. It's sensible for you to try to make every doctor-patient relationship an opportunity for learning and sound decisions. When that's not happening, remember to focus on *your* need: the best medical treatment.

5.

Basic Books for
Active Patients

YOU'VE SEEN YOUR doctor, asked some questions, taken careful notes, and are now ready to begin reading and learning about your medical condition on your own. How do you do it?

This chapter offers a number of practical examples of how various medical reference works are used to find standard medical information. Included are guides, dictionaries, textbooks, manuals, and directories. These resources encompass both the introductory and the comprehensive. They include basic information on symptoms, differential diagnosis, laboratory tests, and much more. It's a good idea to acquaint yourself with these more general sources before you begin to look for journal article titles — something you'll likely want to do later.

The discussion here focuses on printed matter, although the same material is becoming increasingly available on electronic media.

*　　*　　*

WHERE DO YOU START? HOW DO YOU PROCEED?

The story of someone who needed to track down information on breast disease illustrates the typical steps to be taken in researching references and textbooks.

Sally, a teacher in her fifties, was told that her mammogram was suspicious and was referred to a surgeon for evaluation. The same surgeon had two years earlier performed a breast biopsy that revealed she had a benign condition called "sclerosing adenosis." Sally was suddenly concerned that sclerosing adenosis might have increased the risk of breast cancer, and that this might now be what was showing up on the mammogram. Her appointment with the surgeon was more than three weeks away. She had to do something in the meantime to relieve her anxiety.

She first consulted a lay medical dictionary, *Webster's Medical Desk Dictionary*, in her home library. Only by looking up "sclerosing" and "adenosis" separately was she able to learn that the condition is marked by rapidly producing cells and that the tissue they form hardens.

Clearly she was going to need the use of a more comprehensive dictionary. In the library at a local community hospital she soon found, in *Stedman's Medical Dictionary*, a subsection ("adenosis, sclerosing") of the entry for "adenosis," stating: "a nodular benign breast lesion." Although she was relieved that this confirmed the doctor's view that her condition was a benign disease, it did not answer the question about whether this benign disease was likely to turn into breast cancer.

Sally next decided to see what she could find in a medical textbook. Checking the card catalog, she came up with a few choices and selected the one published most recently, *Cecil Textbook of Medicine*. When she looked at the table of contents, however, she was disappointed not to find any references to benign breast disease or sclerosing adenosis. She realized that a general textbook can't cover every medical condition and decided to consult one with a narrower focus.

Going back to the card file, she located *Breast Diseases*, a book containing information on every type of breast disease — malignant or benign. Under a subheading entitled "Pathology of Benign Breast Disorders," sclerosing adenosis is identified under a category called "proliferative without atypia." With the help of *Stedman*'s, she learned that this means, roughly, that the cells proliferate but are not untypical, or irregular. And most important, according to a chart and a discussion in the text, women in this category are *not* part of a group generally at risk for breast cancer. The entry in the textbook was also followed by a number of references, including journal article citations. Had she wanted to locate even more detailed information in medical journals, Sally could easily have started with those references.

With a few hours of modest effort, and no special searching skills, Sally had been able to use books readily accessible in a medical library to considerably relieve her anxiety and make the three-week wait for her appointment with the surgeon tolerable.

When Sally finally did meet with the surgeon, he told her that the suspicious spot on the mammogram was consistent with sclerosing adenosis. Seeing the information in a textbook *and* hearing it from her doctor compounded Sally's faith in the diagnosis, and she left the doctor's office feeling a great burden lifted.

Sally's example provides only a few illustrations of the many basic medical books available to patients. The following sections of this chapter suggest the various classifications of medical reference publications, with specific title examples and details about using them effectively.

POPULAR MEDICAL GUIDES

When you know almost nothing about a medical problem, popular medical guides provide a sensible place to start. Two of the best, available in many public libraries, are the *American Medical Association Family Medical Guide* and the *Mayo Clinic Family Health Book*. Written in nontechnical language, they provide broad descriptions of common diseases and their symptoms as well as information about prevention and self-diagnosis.

For example, the *AMA Guide*'s entry for "hypertension" emphasizes aspects of that condition such as how to change your lifestyle and how to take your own blood pressure. Its discussion of clinical treatment is limited to a few paragraphs pointing out that a doctor will prescribe medication if necessary. The *Mayo Clinic Family Health Book*, however, *does* briefly identify major antihypertensive drug groups.

Popular medical guides explain diseases, treatment processes, and their consequences in easy-to-understand language. For example, an entry for hypertension points out that high blood pressure harms the walls and surfaces of arteries in much the same way that overinflation damages the linings and surfaces of automobile tires. Although there are some differences among popular medical guides, all minimize use of difficult medical terminology, emphasize symptoms and prevention of illness, and tend to be cautious about providing information on treatment.

In addition to these general guides, there are of course hundreds of books written for medical consumers that deal with specific diseases, treatments, or aspects of the treatment process. These books range in quality from excellent (those that few medical specialists would hesitate to recommend to their patients) to potentially hazardous to your health (those based on "junk science" or that tout miracle cures).

You can make a reasonable preliminary judgment of a book's usefulness by determining whether its assertions are documented by references to journal articles and other medical literature, whether it includes a physician as an author (or at least a contributor), and, more generally, whether its tone and use of statistics show respect for scientific methodology. Bear in mind, however, that even the best popular books are likely to be dated by the time they appear in print. They are starting points for more thorough research, not a substitute for it.

Popular guides provide helpful, introductory information about many medical conditions but are not enough to prepare you for substantive searching. For this, you will need sources published for the medical professional.

MEDICAL REFERENCES WRITTEN FOR PROFESSIONALS

Medical Dictionaries

Your principal reference tool will very likely be a medical dictionary. Medical dictionaries written for physicians and published by medical book publishers offer more complete information than their popular counterparts. Most public libraries keep at least one professional medical dictionary in their reference collections, and a medical library will offer several choices. Four useful ones, each of which has been republished in several editions, are *Dorland's Illustrated Medical Dictionary*, *Mosby's Medical Dictionary*, *Stedman's Medical Dictionary*, and *Taber's Cyclopedic Medical Dictionary*. Usually one or more of these should be your starting point for understanding any medical condition in medical terms and will be a resource to which you will return again and again.

No one of these dictionaries is strikingly better than the others. *Dorland's*, *Stedman's*, and *Taber's* contain numerous special sections and appendices covering technical matters such as apothecary and metric dose equivalents and reference values for interpretation of laboratory tests. *Taber's* appendices are especially extensive, including information on topics such as organ donors, hotlines for AIDS, and vitamins. In general, the definitions in *Taber's* tend to be less comprehensive than those in *Dorland's* and *Stedman's*, and its language is less technical. *Mosby's* contains no separate technical sections, but its vocabulary entries are perhaps the easiest to read, often adding a few helpful sentences on diagnosis and treatment. The anatomy charts are excellent in *Dorland's*, *Mosby's*, and *Stedman's*. *Mosby's* is generous with illustrations throughout the text.

Dorland's, *Stedman's*, and *Taber's* contain separate sections that show how medical terms are formed. You learn, for example, that the prefixes "splen-" or "spleno-" mean "of or pertaining to the spleen" and that the suffix "-plenia" means "a condition of the spleen." Similarly, "-itis" means "an inflammation of a particular organ." *Mosby's* includes this information as part of its general vocabulary list. (That is, you simply look up "splen-" and "-itis.")

Although the fundamental organization of any dictionary is alphabetical, these books differ in detail. For example, both *Stedman's* and *Dorland's* list compound words (such as "Marfan's syndrome," a disease from which Abraham Lincoln reputedly suffered) under the noun, in this case "syndrome." Both *Mosby's* and *Taber's* list it under "Marfan's." But a reference to "Marfan's" also appears under the "M" sections of *Stedman's* and *Dorland's*, where it is cross-referenced to "syndrome." Hyphenated or closed compound words, such as "self-awareness" or "afterbirth," appear in normal alphabetical order, that is, under *s* and *a*, respectively.

As you may have gathered, there's a lot to be said for using several dictionaries. One may give you a clue that another omits. As an example of how much information a medical dictionary contains, here's an entry from *Stedman's:*

Marfan's s., a hereditary condition due to congenital changes in the mesodermal and ectodermal tissues, skeletal changes (arachnodactyly, excessive length of extremities, laxness of joints), bilateral ectopia lentis, and vascular defects (particularly aneurysm of the aorta, dissecting or diffuse); iris trans-illumination is marked due to a deficiency of posterior epithelium pigment; autosomal dominant inheritance.

This vocabulary may at first seem alien, but a few of the more familiar words give you a start toward finding out the most important aspect of this condition. Since you probably know *skeletal*, *vascular defects*, and *iris*, you can infer that Marfan's syndrome in some way affects three aspects of the body — its overall framework, including limbs (skeletal); blood vessels (vascular); and eyes (iris).

Looking up unfamiliar words in the same dictionary, you discover that *aneurysm* refers to a dilated artery. The subentries *diffuse* and *dissecting* (the very types mentioned under the definition of Marfan's syndrome) refer to aneurysms that are widespread and in danger of rupturing, respectively.

Aortic is an adjective, but can be treated as in most dictionaries, by finding the noun. It is a "large artery which is the main trunk of the arterial systemic system." By checking two words, you have learned that one serious manifestation of Marfan's syndrome is the rupture of a main blood vessel.

If the word *arachnodactyly* sounds vaguely familiar — reminding you of *arachnophobia* (fear of spiders), you're right. There are two ways you can find this out in *Stedman's* or *Dorland's*. In these dictionaries, you can check a root word list of Greek and Latin words that form the basis of medical terminology. Under *arach-* you would find the reference to a spider or a spider's web. Alternatively, looking up the word *arachnodactyly* itself, you can learn not only its relation to the word *spider* but details of the condition: long hands, fingers, feet, and toes (sometimes), and that it's a regular condition of Marfan's syndrome. (*Mosby's* puts this plainly: "The extremities of individuals with Marfan's syndrome are very long and spiderlike, with greatly extended metacarpals, metatarsals, and phalanges." *Mosby's* also includes a photograph of an individual with Marfan's.)

The entries for Marfan's syndrome in *Dorland's* and *Taber's* are similar to those in *Stedman's*. *Taber's*, for example, reads, "A hereditary syndrome characterized by disorders of connective tissue, bones, eyes, muscles, ligaments, and skeletal structures." Although this entry gives a fair idea of the condition, it does not mention the "vascular defects," as does *Stedman's*. *Mosby's* entry is the longest (over thirty lines) and most informative. It explains, for example, that no specific treatment is advocated for Marfan's, and that physicians usually manage its symptoms by orthotic devices or surgery.

Medical dictionaries can supply the definition of almost any medical term you'll need to know, providing vocabulary used in textbooks and journal articles as well as a general sense of the subject matter. They help provide the first broad brush strokes of the picture that will emerge as your search progresses.

Merck Manual of Diagnosis and Therapy

Although written for health professionals, the *Merck Manual of Diagnosis and Therapy* has for many years occupied a place not only in public and medical libraries but in countless homes as well. Except for a good dictionary, the *Merck Manual*, with its wealth of comprehensive medical information, is likely to be your single most helpful reference.

A compendium of most medical disorders (including dental and psychiatric), the *Merck Manual* describes *in medical terminology* the disorders' causes, symptoms, laboratory tests, diagnosis, treatment, and prognosis. It is arranged by chapters according to the organ or system affected (such as cardiovascular, endocrine, and gastrointestinal) or medical discipline (such as gynecology, pediatrics, and genetics). The opening of each chapter includes a helpful listing of sections and subsections within that chapter. The manual's index is so complete that it would be difficult to miss exact page references for whatever you need to look up. The information itself is equally complete.

For example, in contrast to popular medical guides, the *Merck Manual*'s entry for "hypertension" includes a description of the disease process involved, probable physiological changes that cause high blood pressure, the prevalence of the disease, its symptoms (including retinal changes that can be discovered during an eye examination), the risks of having high blood pressure, and a full description of the generic or trade-name drugs often prescribed, how they work, and their advantages and disadvantages.

Any significant aspect of hypertension, then, from its causes to its various treatments, is fully described in this entry. The example illustrates the extensive information available in the *Merck Manual* and shows why it makes such an excellent starting point for learning the vocabulary and primary characteristics of any medical condition.

The *Merck Manual* is also useful when you need to look up a fairly straightforward condition for immediate information rather than as a prelude to deeper searches. Let's say you simply want to know about an ankle you think may be sprained. The *Merck Manual* entry gives the classifications and treatments of ankle sprains, from mild ones to those that involve a complete tearing of a ligament. It also contains detailed technical information about predisposing factors and how an examination is conducted.

Textbooks of Medicine

For coverage deeper than that found in the *Merck Manual*, you would turn to medical textbooks. Intended for physicians and medical students and written by experts in every field of medicine, they are published in large format and provide expanded and explicit discussion of diseases and their treatment in considerable detail. And what is most important, they generally contain an extensive list of references — the names of publications (books, journal articles, or both) used in the preparation of each entry. These references, which include publishing information (author, title, and date) and a brief description of the article, are an invaluable resource, leading to information from the best journals and the world's leading researchers.

The *Cecil Textbook of Medicine* is one of the best-known and most highly respected medical textbooks. An additional example is *Harrison's Principles of Internal Medicine. Cecil's, Harrison's,* and others are available in university medical libraries and generally in all teaching and community hospitals. They can be found either in the library's reference section or on reserve at the circulation desk, where they can be signed out for in-library use. Some large public libraries in major cities also include these textbooks of medicine in their collections.

Specialty Medical Textbooks

Use specialty medical textbooks when searching less common diseases or when the general medical textbooks give too little information on the condition you're researching. These textbooks offer highly detailed information and often provide the only means of familiarizing oneself thoroughly with the nature of a particular disorder. Recall the example of Sally's search given earlier in the chapter, in which she had to turn to a specialty book on breast diseases because *Cecil's* didn't discuss sclerosing adenosis.

Any medical library contains many volumes of specialty texts. Options for locating them include using the card catalog or an excellent resource that librarians affectionately call the "Brandon list."

Prepared by Alfred N. Brandon and Dorothy R. Hill, this list is published *every other year in the April issue* of the *Bulletin of the Medical Library Association* under the official title, "Selected List of Books and Journals for the Small Medical Library." It contains titles of books recommended in over fifty categories of medicine, such as acquired immunodeficiency syndrome (AIDS), geriatrics, sports medicine, urology, cardiovascular system, and many more. We recommend using it to help locate the names of comprehensive, up-to-date textbooks. (The books listed are current, usually no older than three or four years — often even more recent.) Titles are clearly organized under appropriate headings (Braunwald's *Heart Disease: A Textbook of Cardiovascular Medicine* is listed under the heading "Cardiovascular System," for example). Every library won't have *every* book suggested in the Brandon list. Check the card catalog to see which books you select from the list are in its collection, and when you find one, write down the call number. Go to that section of the library and take the time also to browse through adjacent or nearby books.

Physicians' Desk Reference (PDR)

The *Physicians' Desk Reference (PDR)*, a compendium covering three thousand pharmaceutical products, is a remarkably detailed resource for comprehensive information on prescription and some nonprescription drugs. Keep a medical dictionary nearby when using the *PDR*, to help with unfamiliar words. First, find the name of the drug in the pink pages at the front of the book, in the section called "Product Name Index," using either the brand or generic name (they are cross-referenced). If two page numbers are listed, the first will refer to a four-color section of the *PDR* with a photograph of the pill or medicine container. The second page listed is the one with product information.

The publishers of *PDR* repeat in their book *verbatim and with the same emphasis* the language used in the manufacturer's product information sheet, which must be approved by the Food and Drug Administration (FDA). Each entry describes the use, effects, dosages, and details of how the drug works physiologically and biochemically, and includes warnings, hazards, contraindications (conditions under which it shouldn't be used), side effects, and precautions.

The *PDR* is helpful in other ways. In learning about anti-cancer agents, for example, the entry for levamisole, a drug used in combination with the anti-cancer drug fluorouracil (5FU), describes precisely how it is thought to work in the system against cancer cells. Moreover, references at the end of the article provide names of biomedical journal articles that report on the findings in trial studies using 5FU with levamisole. In this way, anyone wishing to investigate the benefits of using that combination in chemotherapy would have ready citations of articles to read. Although not all drug entries in the *PDR* list references, be sure to check because the references are an invaluable resource.

If a drug prescribed for you comes prepackaged with the product information sheet, this will save you a trip to the *PDR*. If you are receiving thirty pills that the pharmacist took from a much larger bottle, chances are that an information sheet will not be automatically provided. Most pharmacists will be happy to provide you with a package insert if one is available. (This can depend on how a pharmacy receives its shipments from a supplier.) Many people, incidentally, don't realize that pharmacists are excellent information resources. For quick help, check with one of them if you have any question about the specific name or the generic name of a drug or the group of medications into which it falls.

Laboratory Tests

Medical library collections also include comprehensive books about laboratory tests. The *Laboratory Test Handbook* is a good example. Its entries provide details on the interpretation of test results, what a test is commonly given for, other names used for the test (synonyms), specimen instructions, and citations for pertinent references in the biomedical literature.

The *Laboratory Test Handbook* offers three indexes: a *key word index* (look under name of disease, such as "colitis," organ system involved, or syndrome that the test relates to); an *alphabetical index*, which lists test names (and synonyms); and finally, an excellent and very useful *glossary of acronyms and abbreviations*. If you knew only that you had been given an ACT test, for example, you could look in the glossary and learn the full name of the test — "activated clotting time" — then find it in the alphabetical listing.

Medical Specialists Directory

The *Official American Board of Medical Specialists (ABMS) Directory of Board Certified Medical Specialists* is a biographical directory of practicing and retired physicians who are certified by one of twenty-four specialty boards.

Specialty board certification guarantees that a physician has trained and passed examinations in a specific area of medicine, going beyond the basic training and examinations required to receive a medical degree. Specialists often study for as many as eight years before they become practitioners in their field. The directory provides essential information about ABMS board-certified medical specialists anywhere in the United States. Information includes date of birth, name of medical school, places of internship and residencies, fellowship (postdoctoral) training, type of medical practice, professional associations, and current appointments (academic and hospital). "Residency" refers to postgraduate specialty training. Subspecialty training usually takes place in a fellowship program following residency.

Published in four volumes, the *ABMS Directory* can be used in two ways: to find a specific physician in the alphabetical master index at the end of volume four, or to search for specialists listed in a particular geographical area (state and city). Directions for using this directory are unusually clear and appear in the opening pages of each of the four volumes.

A sample entry (see Figure 5-1) shows that Susan E. Brextin, who was born in 1938 in Cleveland, Ohio, received a doctor of medicine degree (M.D.) at Jefferson Medical College in 1965 (some entries indicate D.O., for doctor of osteopathy). After one year's internship at Temple University Hospital, she did her surgical residency at Thomas Jefferson University Hospital from 1968 to 1972. Later, she obtained subspecialty training in vascular surgery at Temple during 1972–1973. She has hospital appointments at Good Samaritan and Johns Hopkins, both in Baltimore. She is a member of the American Medical Association (AMA), a Fellow of the American College of Surgeons (FACS), and is in solo full-time private practice.

A Biographical Sketch

All biographies include type of specialty, and subspecialty if applicable, and years of certification, subcertification, recertification and time limitation as appropriate.

A full biography will tell you the specialist's year of birth, date of medical degree and the university conferring the degree. The entry will show the doctor's hospital affiliations starting with his or her residency up to the present time, the national medical societies to which he or she belongs and the type of practice the doctor maintains, such as private practice solo or medical administration. The sketch ends with the doctor's address and phone/fax number.

In the case of some physicians, a full entry is not included. This may be because the physician has been recently certified and has not yet had an opportunity to submit full information or because the doctor has not responded to requests for more information. If a physician's address is not known, he or she is placed under the city of the last known address. If the last known address is unavailable, the specialist is placed under "Address Unavailable" after each specialty. The following is an example of a full biographical sketch.

Specialist's Name

Subspecialty & Dates

Certification (Cert),
Recertification (R) & Dates

Medical School

BALTIMORE

●BREXTIN, Susan E.

Internship

Birth Year & Place

●Cert S 76 R85-95. ●(PdS)87-97. ●b 38
Cleveland OH. MD ●Jefferson Med College
65.

Residency

Hospital Appointments

●Int 65-66 (Temple U Hosp Philadelphia)

Fellowship

● Res Surg 68-69 Res 70-72 (both at
Thomas Jefferson U Hosp Philadelphia)

Academic Appointments

Type of Practice
FT = Full-Time
PT = Part-Time

●Fell PdS 72-73 (Temple U Hosp
Philadelphia).

Professional Memberships
(F) = Fellow

●Att Phys 74-86(Good Samaritan Hosp,
Baltimore) Chief Surg 87- (Meml Hosp
Baltimore).●Instr 84-86 (U Md) Prof Surg
87- (Johns Hopkins U). ●AMA-ACS(F)-
ISCS.●PT-Salr Hosp Clin, PT- Acad Fac.

Primary Office Address,
Phone & Fax

Secondary Office Address,
Street, City, State & Zip

●2 Elm St #502 21210 (410)555-1212 Fax:
(410)555-1213 ●48 Grant Ave Annapolis
MD 21403.

*Note: This is a hypothetical listing and not intended for actual reference.
NOTATIONS USED

Certification
Certification is indicated by the abbreviation "Cert" followed by the letter code for the specialty and the last two digits of the year in which the certificate was issued.
Cert S 79 .Certified in **Surgery** in 1979.

Subcertification
Subcertification is indicated by the letter code for the subspecialty contained in parenthesis followed by the last two digits of the year in which the subcertification was issued.
Cert S 79 (PdS) 82 Subcertified in **Pediatric Surgery** in 1982.

Recertification
Recertification is indicated by the letter "R" and the last two digits of the year in which the recertification was issued.
Cert S 79, R88 Certified in Surgery in 1979, **Recertified** in 1988.
Cert S 59 (PdS)75, R84 Certified in Surgery in 1959, subcertification of Pediatric Surgery in 1975, **Recertified in Pediatric Surgery in 1984.**

In 1987, the American Board of Internal Medicine offered a special recertification examination noted as:
AAIM/R87 Advanced Achievement in Internal Medicine.

Time Limited Certification
Some Boards that issue time-limited certificates also indicate the year of expiration. This is noted as:
Cert FP 85-92 Certified in 1985 for the period 1985 through 1992.
Cert FP 82, R89-96 Originally certified in 1982, **Recertified for the period 1989 through 1996.**

Names of diplomates who have not recertified within the time limit are not listed in the directory with one exception. Names of diplomates of the American Board of Thoracic Surgery who have not recertified within the time limit are included within the following notation:
Cert TS 78NR Certified in 1978, **Not Recertified.**

Figure 5-1. Sample entry from *ABMS Directory*.

An additional feature of the *ABMS Directory* is the listing, in each volume, of medical schools by state. This is a good reference for locating a nearby university hospital.

In general, membership on the faculty of a university hospital indicates the doctor's association with an environment in touch with the latest technical advances. Also, since university hospitals are usually major referral centers in an area, they generally have the most experience and are sent the toughest cases. Specialists with the *closest connection* to a university hospital (as shown under "current hospital appointment" — look for a "U" to signify "university") have an *academic appointment* to the faculty of the associated medical school. This is indicated by an academic title such as "professor" or "associate professor."

One of the most helpful features is the section describing specialties and subspecialties. Each entry summarizes in explicit language what the specialist and subspecialist actually does in a medical practice. For example, under "Anesthesiology":

> The anesthesiologist is a physician-specialist who, following medical school graduation and at least four years of postgraduate training, has the principal task of providing pain relief and maintenance, or restoration, of a stable condition during and immediately following an operation, an obstetric or diagnostic procedure.

This description continues for several lines, providing more details and examples of the anesthesiologist's functions and skills.

The *ABMS Directory* is the best resource available for getting leads on well-qualified specialist physicians. Note, however, that there are well over one hundred other groups that certify "specialists." Some non-ABMS certifying bodies have rigorous standards; others do not. It may take careful questioning and perhaps a call to a state health department to discover a particular group's standards. Note also that some non-ABMS specialty names are quite similar to ABMS names. For example, while "Anesthesiology" is an ABMS-recognized specialty, "Anesthesia" is not. For a fast check on whether a physician is board certified or whether a subspecialty is recognized by the ABMS, you can call an ABMS hotline (1-800-776-2378). If a physician or specialty is not listed, the ABMS operator will usually be able to provide a phone number for the board to contact for more information.

LIBRARIES

From the National Library of Medicine in Bethesda, Maryland, to a community library in Kearney, Nebraska, all the libraries in this country are equipped to help you start learning about your medical condition. Even small public libraries keep basic medical references in their collection, and that's a beginning.

Some public libraries, particularly the larger ones, are well provided with resources to handle many consumer health questions. If you wish, you can explore public libraries first. But if you are involved in a deeper-level search of biomedical literature, many of your questions and information needs can be met only by the resources available in a medical library.

Librarians

Specialized medical libraries can be complicated to navigate. If you need any help in finding your way around or locating information, be sure to ask the librarian. (Just keep in mind that you may sometimes have to wait a short while until the librarian can give you full attention.) Reference librarians serve as superb support systems and are well versed in the vocabulary of medicine, search processes, and the content of the library collection — they're required to hold advanced degrees in library science.

Librarians prefer that you ask specific, rather than general, questions. For example, if you want information about a childhood illness, don't ask for pediatric journals but rather for information about the specific disease, if you know it, or at least the general type of medical condition. There's no need to be afraid of appearing not to know medical terminology. Just articulate your question clearly, so that a librarian can narrow the search and help you find what you want more quickly. "All anybody has to do is ask an intelligent question and smile," says one medical reference librarian, "and we're ready to drop everything and help."

GENERAL CATEGORIES OF LIBRARIES

The National Library of Medicine and Regional Libraries

This country's principal medical library is the National Library of Medicine (NLM). Access to many of its resources is made available nationwide through the National Network of Libraries of Medicine (NN/LM) and its eight regional libraries, located in New York, Baltimore, Chicago, Omaha, Houston, Seattle, Los Angeles, and Farmington, Connecticut. Regional libraries handle requests for medical literature not available locally and pass requests they cannot fill on to the NLM. (See Appendix A for a full listing of states included in each region and the address and phone number of each regional medical library.)

If you have a question about locating some medical literature, you can contact your regional library by calling 1-800-338-7657. Once you're connected, press "1" and you will be automatically transferred to the regional library in the area from which you're calling. Ask to speak with a reference librarian. Some librarians will help you directly, and others will give you the names of medical libraries in their referral system that are closer to where you live.

Academic Medical Libraries

Dedicated to scholarship in the medical sciences, academic medical libraries are almost always libraries connected with a medical college or university. They have the largest collections of reference and textbooks, medical journals, and access to computerized databases. Call first to make sure they are open to the public. These libraries sometimes serve only staff and faculty members (generally in private universities), depending on individual policy. If you do have access to an academic library, try to take advantage of it.

Teaching and Community Hospital Libraries

Teaching and community hospital libraries hold collections of medical science books and journals that are smaller than those at university hospitals, but these libraries generally maintain a very strong core collection of biomedical literature. In recent years, many of them have made substantial efforts to serve members of the public, such as providing individual help in finding reference material on the shelves, offering free use and instruction on searching medical bibliographic indexes (both print and electronic), and setting up booths in shopping malls from which questions are forwarded to the library. Policies about public use differ among libraries, although most are open to everyone. Naturally, it's wise to call a library before making the trip to use it.

Public Libraries

Public libraries shouldn't be overlooked. In major cities, such as Boston, public libraries have extensive collections of biomedical literature. Central libraries in smaller urban areas often keep strong collections of medical reference books, including dictionaries, medical encyclopedias, and textbooks. Some of the material they keep, however, is oriented more toward the casual health consumer than someone seriously researching medical options.

Note that many public libraries have installed computers with publication indexes that can easily be used to locate magazine and journal articles about a given disease. Be aware, however, that generally only a very few of the medical journals that are indexed by the NLM are catalogued in the public library indexes. They do, though, include major medical journals, such as the *New England Journal of Medicine*.

CONSUMER HEALTH INFORMATION RESOURCES
LIBRARIES

An additional class of libraries includes those devoted exclusively to the medical consumer. Although generally affiliated with hospitals, these information centers are usually designated as separate entities that include instruction and other services, as well as a library collection — all open or available to the public. A well-known example is the Planetree Health Resource Center, with locations in both in San Francisco and San Jose. Another is the Health Education Center in Pittsburgh.

Consumer health information resource libraries exist in many communities across the United States. All of them provide a good starting point for researching a condition, and some offer access to professional-level literature.

THE VALUE OF GOOD RESEARCH TOOLS

"If you ever find yourself in a similar situation," says one patient who was unexpectedly hospitalized, "the first thing to do is tell your family to forgo the flowers and magazines and bring you, instead, a good medical dictionary."

You needn't — and shouldn't — wait until an emergency to recognize the value of good medical research tools. Those discussed in this chapter can provide substantial information upon which all your ensuing research efforts will build. You can decide whether you'll use some of these references often enough to warrant purchasing them. A good dictionary and the *Merck Manual* are affordable.

Only a few of the great number of medical references available are listed here. The main point to remember is that almost any kind of health-related information you want is available in medical and, to some extent, public libraries. (In addition, many of these materials are beginning to appear on CD-ROM.) Understanding how to use various resources reviewed here will make searches in journal articles, as discussed in the next chapter, far more productive.

6.

How to Launch Effective Searches

THE VERY LATEST medical information is far too new to be included in medical textbooks and often too narrowly publicized to have been noticed by your doctor. To find out about it, you have to read medical journals written by and for physicians and scientists. These journals are where professionals on the cutting edge of research communicate with each other and with doctors who will sooner or later put new knowledge into practice.

This chapter will introduce you to the principal printed reference tools needed to locate medical journal articles — *Index Medicus* and its companion aids to medical literature searches. You'll find that searching this medical index is not very different from searching a magazine article index, such as the *Readers' Guide to Periodical Literature*. The concept and the techniques are much the same, even if the subject matter is more technical. The following chapter will offer suggestions on understanding the kinds of articles to be found there.

*   *   *

INDEX MEDICUS

Index Medicus is the most comprehensive print index to the world's biomedical literature. Well over one hundred years old, it's published by the National Library of Medicine (NLM).

Index Medicus, appearing monthly, consists of two softcover volumes the size of metropolitan telephone directories. It indexes articles from more than three thousand medical journals. Its citations, indexed separately by subject and by author, consist of the name of an article's first or sole author, the article title, the title of the journal in which it appears, and the information needed to locate the article (date, volume, issue number, and pages). There's usually a lag of about three months from the time an article is first published to when it appears in *Index Medicus*. *Index Medicus* is also published annually under the title *Cumulated Index Medicus*, filling seventeen volumes. The monthly and annual versions are identically organized. You will find *Index Medicus* primarily in libraries connected to medical schools and large hospitals, and perhaps in larger public libraries.

NLM also publishes a shorter version, the *Abridged Index Medicus (AIM)*, also cumulated annually as *Cumulated Abridged Index Medicus*. *AIM* can be found in the libraries of most community hospitals and many public libraries. Its organization is very similar to that of its full-sized counterpart, but it indexes articles from only 119 English-language medical journals judged most useful for physicians and researchers. This is an impressive number of journals in its own right but amounts to only a small fraction of the total medical literature.

MEDICAL SUBJECT HEADINGS (MeSH)

We'll begin with searches by subject, which are more complex than those by author.

Searching any index is easy if you know the exact term you're looking for — in this case, the headings used in *Index Medicus* to classify articles on the question you're researching. Unfortunately, you may not know that. If you're just starting out, you probably will not. Even if you've taken careful notes on what your doctor told you, he or she may not have mentioned some point that you'll find to be important or may have used a colloquial term rather than a technical one — for example, "high blood pressure" rather than "hypertension."

Fortunately, *Index Medicus* provides a companion volume (updated annually) called *Medical Subject Headings* (commonly abbreviated to *MeSH*). *MeSH* is divided into two parts. The first part, called the "Alphabetic List," is just what it sounds like: an alphabetically ordered list of subject headings used in *Index Medicus*, including cross-references. The second part of *MeSH* is called "Tree Structures," and we'll return to it in due course.

Even if you're fairly sure you know the exact term you want to look up in *Index Medicus*, it's still a good idea to consult at least the *MeSH* alphabetic list. Doing this will help you see your problem in its proper medical context and may suggest important literature in related fields. The librarians who developed *MeSH* anticipated these needs and built two kinds of cross-references into *MeSH*. The first is indicated by "see," as in "Blood Pressure, High, see Hypertension." This means that "high blood pressure" and "hypertension" are synonyms. The second is indicated by "see related," as in "Hypertension see related Vascular Resistance." "Vascular resistance" is related to "hypertension" but not a synonym for it. For terms with multiple cross-references, "see" is shortened to the code symbol "X," and "see related" to "XR." (Before 1991, a third cross-reference phrase, "see under," referred to a term's place in a hierarchy, but it is no longer used.) Figure 6-1 shows an excerpt from the *MeSH* alphabetic list of subject headings.

The indexers who assign subject headings to journal articles for inclusion in *Index Medicus* always use the *most specific subject heading* available for each indexable concept. This means that articles about "Phenobarbital" will be found under that heading rather than the broader heading "Anticonvulsants." Hence articles listed in *Index Medicus* under "Anticonvulsants" deal with (a) anticonvulsants in general and (b) anticonvulsants that don't have their own subject headings in *MeSH*. This means that to find all the articles you want under a broad subject heading, you may have to check under several specific ones.

Hypertension
C14.907.489+
see related
        Antihypertensive Agents
        Vascular Resistance
X   Blood Pressure, High
XR   Blood Pressure

Hypertension-Edema-Proteinuria Gestosis see Gestosis, EPH

Hypertension, Goldblatt see Hypertension, Renovascular

Hypertension, Malignant
C14.907.489.330

Hypertension, Portal
C6.552.494+   C14.907.489.430+
see related
        Portasystemic Shunt, Surgical

Hypertension, Pulmonary
C14.907.489.531+
see related
        Pulmonary Heart Disease
X   Ayerza's Syndrome

Hypertension, Pulmonary, of Newborn, Persistent see Persistent Fetal Circulation
    Syndrome

Hypertension, Renal
C12.777.419.331+   C14.907.489.631+

Hypertension, Renovascular
C12.777.419.331.490   C14.907.489.631.485
84; was see under HYPERTENSION, RENAL 1979-83
X   Hypertension, Goldblatt
XR   Renal Artery Obstruction

Figure 6-1. Subject headings related to hypertension as they appear in
the **MeSH** alphabetic list. Current subject headings appear in large
type; synonyms (in small type) are cross-referenced by "see" to current subject headings. Code numbers indicate where a subject heading appears within the hierachical **MeSH** tree structure, which
follows the alphabetic list.

Because of the sheer quantity of medical literature, you'll more
often be concerned with narrowing a search than broadening one.
You'll appreciate *MeSH*'s orientation toward specificity when

you're searching for articles related to a medical condition for which there are thousands of entries. Take AIDS, for example, a subject heading that directs you to "see Acquired Immunodeficiency Syndrome." The 1993 *Cumulated Index Medicus* contains twenty-five pages of entries under "Acquired Immunodeficiency Syndrome," each page containing well over one hundred citations. Most of these will be unrelated to any analysis of treatment options — for example, reports on funding for AIDS research or statistics on the spread of AIDS in Asia. If your specific interest, however, is "Kaposi's Sarcoma," one of the secondary cancers associated with AIDS, look for material under "Sarcoma, Kaposi's." In short, *Index Medicus*'s cross-references help you expand searches; its tightly defined categories help you narrow them.

MeSH Subheadings

Before leaving the *MeSH* Alphabetic List, note a special set of classification terms called "subheadings." The terms *subject headings* and *subheadings* sound similar, but they perform entirely different functions. We've been talking about *subject headings;* that is, terms used to categorize a condition, treatment, or technique about which an article is written. Subheadings appear *under* subject headings in *Index Medicus*, but they are not simply second-order categories. Their function is to provide a common terminology pertinent to many subject headings — for example, the *subheading* "Adverse Effects" appears under virtually all drug-related *subject headings*.

Altogether, there are eighty such subheadings that appear under subject headings throughout *Index Medicus*. These subheadings are listed in the first volumes of both the monthly and annual versions. (They are omitted from the monthly editions of the *Abridged Index Medicus*.)

The most obvious use of subheadings is in narrowing a search. For example, if your immediate interest is confined to research on drugs used in treating prostate cancer (whose subject heading is "Prostatic Neoplasms"), check the article citations and *MeSH* cross references under the subheading "Drug Therapy," but ignore the subheadings "Surgery" or "Radiotherapy." Conversely, subheadings may be used to broaden your search perspective. For example, if you had assumed that the only treatment for prostate cancer is surgery, simply noting that the subject heading "Prostatic Neoplasms" includes articles under the subheadings "Drug Therapy" and "Radiotherapy" might suggest other options.

MeSH Tree Structures

In addition to its alphabetic list of subject headings, *MeSH* contains a series of hierarchical listings called "Tree Structures." Tree structures can be very useful in helping determine appropriate subject headings for your search.

The tree structures contain all *MeSH* subject headings placed under one or more of fifteen very broad categories, such as "Anatomy," "Diseases," and "Chemicals and Drugs." These categories, which might be thought of as trunks of trees, branch into their own hierarchies of increasingly specific terms. The function of tree structures, therefore, is to help you to place the subject you are researching into a broader context (and sometimes more than one). Tree structures can be especially helpful when you are bogged down with a term that isn't yielding any promising citations in *Index Medicus*. (Note that this is just the opposite of the problem of trying to narrow your search to a manageable number of entries under a much-studied condition like AIDS.)

For example, Judy Logan, a reference librarian in a New England academic medical library, recalls how the use of *MeSH* tree structures helped clarify a search problem for a young woman whose sister had just given birth to a baby diagnosed with Lutembacher's syndrome.

> She had found "Lutembacher's Syndrome" listed as a subject heading in the *MeSH* book. When she looked in the appropriate volume of *Index Medicus*, the young woman discovered that only one reference was listed. I suggested that we look in *MeSH* and write down the tree number that appears just below the subject heading "Lutembacher's Syndrome."

That number was C14.240.400.560.375.518. Turning to the C14 subsection of the tree structure, Logan and the young woman found a page like Figure 6-2 below, whose main heading is "Cardiovascular Diseases (C14)." One of that broad heading's main subcategories is "Cardiovascular Abnormalities" (C14.240), which branches into increasingly specific subject headings: "Heart Defects, Congenital" (C14.240.400), "Heart Septal Defects," (C14.240.400.560), "Heart Septal Defects, Atrial" (C14.240.400.560.375), and, at last, "Lutembacher's Syndrome." By searching under the subject heading ("Heart Septal Defects, Atrial") that appears just *above* Lutembacher's syndrome, the young woman found a number of helpful citations for articles that dealt with Lutembacher's syndrome as one example of a broader, but not unmanageably broad, set of problems.

Cardiovascular Diseases	C14		
Cardiovascular Abnormalities (Non MeSH)	C14.240	C16.131.240	
Arterio-Arterial Fistula	C14.240.110	C14.907.933.	C16.131.240.
		C23.439.850.	
Arteriovenous Malformations	C14.240.150	C14.907.150	C16.131.240.
Arteriovenous Fistula	C14.240.150.125	C14.907.150	C14.907.933.
		C16.131.240	C23.439.850
Cerebral Arteriovenous Malformations	C14.240.150.295	C10.228.140.	C14.907.150.
		C14.907.253.	C16.131.240
Heart Defects, Congenital	C14.240.400	C14.280.400.	C16.131.240.
Aortic Coarctation	C14.240.400.90	C14.280.400.	C16.131.240.
Cor Triatriatum	C14.240.400.200	C14.280.400.	C16.131.240.
Coronary Vessel Anomalies	C14.240.400.210	C14.280.400.	C16.131.240.
Crisscross Heart	C14.240.400.220	C14.280.400.	C16.131.240.
Dextrocardia	C14.240.400.280	C14.280.400.	C16.131.240.
		C16.131.810.	
Ductus Arteriosus, Patent	C14.240.400.340	C14.280.400.	C16.131.240.
Ebstein's Anomaly	C14.240.400.395	C14.280.400.	C16.131.240.
Eisenmenger Complex	C14.240.400.450	C14.280.400.	C16.131.240.
Heart Septal Defects	C14.240.400.560	C14.280.400.	C16.131.240.
Aortopulmonary Septal Defect	C14.240.400.560.98	C14.280.400.	C16.131.240.
Endocardial Cushion Defects	C14.240.400.560.350	C14.280.400.	C16.131.240.
Heart Septal Defects, Atrial	C14.240.400.560.375	C14.280.400.	C16.131.240.
Lutembacher's Syndrome	C14.240.400.560.375.518	C14.280.400.	C16.131.240.
Trilogy of Fallot	C14.240.400.560.375.702	C14.280.400.	C16.131.240.
Heart Septal Defects, Ventricular	C14.240.400.560.540	C14.280.400.	C16.131.240.
Hypoplastic Left Heart Syndrome	C14.240.400.625	C14.280.400.	C16.131.240.
Levocardia	C14.240.400.701	C14.280.400.	C16.131.240.
		C16.131.810.	

Figure 6-2. The hierarchical nature of the **MeSH** tree structure is illustrated by the appearance of "Lutembacher's Syndrome" as one of the smaller branches of tree whose main trunk is "C14: Cardiovascular Diseases." The numbers that appear in smaller type on the right hand side of the page indicate other parts of the **MeSH** tree structure where many entries, including "Lutembacher's Syndrome," also appear.

Searches That Can Be Tricky

You may have to rely on trial and error to find some subject headings. For example, it can sometimes be tricky to look up a drug in *MeSH*. "Prozac," the trade name for an antidepressant, is not a subject heading, but problems in finding it can easily be remedied if you are in a medical library. Ask the reference librarian for the generic name of Prozac (or any other drug for which you only know the trade name). Or check any drug reference book, such as *Physicians' Desk Reference*, that lists both the generic and trade names. In this case, Prozac is the trade name for fluoxetine, which *is* an alphabetic subject heading and is listed in the tree structures section of *MeSH* under the broader heading "Antidepressive Agents."

You'll learn most of the other terms peculiar to your search as you go along. For example, the first time you look under the subject heading "Cancer," you may be surprised that the only subheading is "Care Facilities." But the fine print just below reads "Cancer see Neoplasms." *MeSH* lists almost all the articles pertaining to cancer under the larger heading "Neoplasms," for cancer is a type of neoplasm. Keeping this in mind, you won't have any trouble finding articles about, say, colon cancer. They'll be listed under "Colonic Neoplasms." Specific types of colon cancer, such as adenocarcinoma, also appear as subject headings. The main point to remember is that you don't have to know all of this, or even any of it, in advance. By using *MeSH* systematically, moving back and forth between its alphabetic list and its tree structures as needed, you can soon identify the subject headings worth searching. Almost as important, considering the vast amount of medical literature produced each year, you'll soon develop confidence in decisions about which subject headings you can safely ignore.

MeSH citations are clear, and you'll have no difficulty understanding them. If you're not sure how to decipher the abbreviation for a journal title, check a supplement to *Index Medicus*, the *List of Journals Indexed (LJI)*, which is found in the January (unbound) volume of *Index Medicus* for the current year or in Volume One of its annual cumulation.

PERMUTED MEDICAL SUBJECT HEADINGS

Another useful tool is the supplemental publication *Permuted Medical Subject Headings. Permuted MeSH* takes all significant words from every subject heading and lists them separately, showing under each an indented list of all the headings in which that word appears. For example, Figure 6-3 shows two entries from *Permuted MeSH*, one for "Acquired," the other for "AIDS." Note that the "Acquired" entry includes many terms that have nothing to do with AIDS, such as "Ear Deformities, Acquired." The "AIDS" entry includes a few terms that have nothing to do with "Acquired Immunodeficiency Syndrome," such as "Audio-Visual Aids."

Permuted MeSH is especially useful when you can remember only one word of a subject heading. Its introduction offers as an example "Idiopathic Hypertrophic Subvalvular Stenosis," a subject heading of which a reader might recall only the single word "stenosis" (surely a forgivable lapse in memory). By checking "Stenosis," one finds the whole term. *Permuted MeSH* may also suggest new search ideas. For example, under a word like "child" you'll find possibly useful entries like "Mother-Child Relations." This entry would not have been suggested by either the alphabetic list or the *MeSH* tree structures.

Permuted MeSH is published in support of searches within MEDLINE, an electronic, expanded version of *Index Medicus* described in chapter 10. Therefore you're more likely to find it near computer terminals than shelved with *Index Medicus*. Ask the librarian to help you locate a copy.

REVIEW ARTICLES

The simplest way to find those articles most likely to be informative is to concentrate your search, at least at first, on review articles, which are broad, well-documented surveys of the existing literature on a subject. This type of journal article lists all the bibliographic sources its author has used, with references. They are gold mines of leads to pertinent research and can often save time.

Acquired

Acquired Immunodeficiency Syndrome
Anemia, Hemolytic, Acquired see Anemia, Hemolytic
Anemia, Hemolytic, Idiopathic Acquired see Anemia, Hemolytic, Autoimmune
Aphasia, Acquired
Community-Acquired Infections
Dyslexia, Acquired
Ear Deformities, Acquired
Epidermolysis Bullosa, Acquired see Epidermolysis Bullosa Acquisita
Feline Acquired Immunodeficiency Syndrome
Fetal Immunity, Maternally-Acquired see Immunity, Maternally-Acquired
Foot Deformities, Acquired
Hand Deformities, Acquired
Immunity, Maternally-Acquired
Immunodeficiency Syndrome, Acquired see Acquired Immunodeficiency
    Syndrome
Immunologic Deficiency Syndrome, Acquired see Acquired Immunodeficiency
    Syndrome
Joint Deformities, Acquired
Maternally-Acquired Immunity see Immunity, Maternally-Acquired
Murine Acquired Immunodeficiency Syndrome
Neonatal Immunity, Maternally-Acquired see Immunity, Maternally-Acquired
Nose Deformities, Acquired
Reading Disability, Acquired see Dyslexia, Acquired
Simian Acquired Immunodeficiency Syndrome

AIDS

AIDS see Acquired Immunodeficiency Syndrome
AIDS Antibodies see HIV Antibodies
AIDS Antigens see HIV Antigens
AIDS-Associated Lymphoma see Lymphoma, AIDS-Related
AIDS-Associated Nephropathy
AIDS Dementia Complex
AIDS Encephalopathy see AIDS Dementia Complex
AIDS, Feline see Feline Acquired Immunodeficiency Syndrome
AIDS, Murine see Murine Acquired Immunodeficiency Syndrome
AIDS-Related Complex
AIDS-Related Lymphoma see Lymphoma, AIDS-Related
AIDS-Related Opportunistic Infections
AIDS Seroconversion see HIV Seropositivity
AIDS Serodiagnosis
AIDS Serology see AIDS Serodiagnosis
AIDS Seropositivity see HIV Seropositivity
AIDS, Simian see Simian Acquired Immunodeficiency Syndrome
AIDS Vaccines
AIDS Virus see HIV-1
AIDS Virus Receptors see Receptors, HIV
Audio-Visual Aids
Communication Aids for Disabled
Communication Aids for Handicapped see Communication Aids for Disabled
Feline AIDS see Feline Acquired Immunodeficiency Syndrome
Hearing Aids
Lymphoma, AIDS-Related
Murine AIDS see Murine Acquired Immunodeficiency Syndrome
Opportunistic infections, AIDS-Related see AIDS-Related Opportunistic
    Infections
Pharmaceutic Aids
Sensory Aids
Simian AIDS see Simian Acquired Immunodificiency Syndrome
Simian AIDS Retrovirus see Retroviruses Type D, Simian

Figure 6-3. These are **Permuted Medical Subject Headings** entries under both "acquired" and "AIDS," identifying every **MeSH** subject heading in which either word appears. **Permuted MeSH** can be used to locate any subject heading if you know even one word of the full heading.

Their critiques may also help you judge the worth of articles you've previously located but would like to know more about.

Each month's full *Index Medicus* includes a section called *Bibliography of Medical Reviews* (*BMR*). This contains citations for review articles only. The annual cumulation covers the most recent five years. Moreover, review articles within the subject section of *Index Medicus* are easily identified by a parenthetical notation to references. For example, in a 1994 *Index Medicus*, the following citation appears under the subject heading "Hypertension," subheading "Drug Therapy":

Selected factors that influence responses to antihypertensives. Choosing therapy for the uncomplicated patient. Carter BL, et al. Arch Fam Med 1994 Jun; 3(6):528–36 (87 ref.)

The concluding parenthetical note tells you that this is a review article that cites 87 references — strongly suggesting that it is a comprehensive overview of its subject. You could locate and read any of these you decide might be pertinent.

SEARCHES BY AUTHOR AND THE *SCIENCE CITATION INDEX*

The techniques of searching *Index Medicus* by author require little explanation. For articles with multiple authors, *Index Medicus* lists the full citation of an article only under the principal author, but it lists up to ten other authors, cross-referenced to the principal one. For example, "Lang P see Brandt B" means that Lang is a coauthor of an article over which Brandt's name appears first. Under "Brandt B" you would see the complete citation.

A search by author can be useful for either of two reasons. First, an author of an interesting article may have written other articles that you'll find equally pertinent. You could locate them under their appropriate subject headings, but checking the author's name is easier. Second, you may want to check out the credentials of a physician who's been recommended to you as a specialist. A publication record is one indicator of standing in his or her field.

This seems an appropriate place to mention another index, not part of the NLM family of medical research publications, that can contribute to a search. This is the *Science Citation Index* (*SCI*), published by the Institute for Scientific Information, Philadelphia. The *SCI* indexes literature in science, medicine, agriculture, technology, and the social sciences. It shows how often an article has been cited in subsequent scientific and medical literature and thus provides, at least for articles over two or three years old, a fairly reliable indication of that article's importance in the eyes of other researchers. (News notices and most book reviews are omitted, so the citations show an older article's actual use or influence.)

The *SCI* also provides a way of locating other relevant articles. Suppose you've been impressed by an article published by someone named Able in 1990. A check of the *SCI* shows that it was indeed cited repeatedly in 1992, 1993, and 1994, suggesting that Able's peers share your opinion of its value. Moreover, a check of the authors who cited Able leads you to later articles by Baker, Charles, and others that you might otherwise have missed. Also, like *MeSH*, the *SCI* provides a way of doing subject searches through its *Permuterm Subject Index* (*PSI*).

In general, the *SCI* is a tool for an advanced stage of your researches. This doesn't mean that it's difficult to use, merely that you're unlikely to need it until you've already done considerable work in *Index Medicus*.

CHOOSING AND LOCATING ARTICLES

When you are searching *Index Medicus*, the titles of articles provide the only clue about how pertinent they are. Many of them can be eliminated out of hand, because they clearly bear no relevance to the subject. Study the title carefully, recognizing that the scientists and doctors who write the articles assign *explicit* titles. Their obligation is to make the title as clear as possible for the sake of the indexers and readers who are familiar with medical literature. Some titles may be long and contain a few unfamiliar words (so keep a medical dictionary handy). But usually the title will be nearly self-explanatory, as in "Fertility outcome following tubal pregnancy."

The introduction to *Index Medicus* includes several pages of information on getting access to the articles whose citations you locate. In practice, if the library you're using does not have a copy of the journal you're looking for, you should simply ask its librarian to advise you on obtaining it through interlibrary loan. Some medical libraries may offer to obtain a copy for you; others don't have the staff to serve outside patrons. In either case, the librarian will know the best way for you to get an article.

A number of commercial document delivery services exist, and a source of information on them is listed in this book's bibliography. One especially extensive service is operated by the Colorado Alliance of Research Libraries (CARL). It maintains a regularly updated database called UnCover, which contains well over five million items (not exclusively medical). You can arrange for delivery in a variety of ways, including both hard copy and e-mail. Charges vary, depending in part on copyright fees, but are competitive. For more information, contact CARL's subsidiary, the UnCover Company, 3801 East Florida Ave., Suite 200, Denver, CO 80210, (303) 758-3030.

SEARCH STRATEGIES SUMMARIZED

Effective searching is as much an art as a science, but a systematic approach will make your search more productive. Keeping the following points in mind will help you develop good search strategies:

• Be prepared. If possible, bring to the library a written list of names and terms, ideally based on your talks with your doctor, that you expect to be the subjects of your search.

• Be patient. Rather than just plunging into *Index Medicus*, consult *MeSH* for the appropriate *subject headings* under which to look for titles.

• Be thorough. Look under *subheadings* for ideas on what aspect of your subject to consider.

- Use *MeSH* tree structures to broaden or refine your search.
- Use *Permuted Medical Subject Headings* to see all the headings in which the name of your subject appears.
- When you get ready to read articles, give first priority to review articles. In many cases, you may have to go no further. If you do need to go further, their references will provide valuable leads.

It's appropriate that the developers of *Index Medicus* chose to call its principal support tool *MeSH*. It's a nice acronym, conveying as it does a sense of integration and of parts functioning together harmoniously. The logical skills you develop and the medical terminology you acquire while using *MeSH* and *Index Medicus* will stand you in good stead during every stage of your search for the best treatment, whether you're using reference materials or assimilating comments by your physicians.

7.

How to Learn from
Medical Journals

YOUR MOST VALUABLE source of detailed information on current medical treatments will be professional scientific journal articles. This chapter discusses the characteristics of those articles, including their purpose and organization. It suggests how to find the sum and substance of what you need from them.

The most important article Suzanne (one of this book's authors) ever read was a study entitled "Results of Surgical Excision of One to 13 Hepatic Metastases in 98 Consecutive Patients," written by John Peter Minton, M.D., Ph.D. The flat, colorless words of this title guided her to a surgeon who saved her mother's life.

Hidden beneath the undramatic title and the detached, objective language of the article was exactly the kind of factual, unbiased information that Suzanne needed to help her make a decision. She knew from her husband, a scientist, that doctors and scientists use journal articles to communicate new information to each other. Unlike popular magazine or newspaper articles, which may be oversimplified, misleading, or even incorrect, these articles are bound by the rules of scientific investigation, which demand objectivity and supportable evidence.

WHY JOURNAL ARTICLES ARE HIGHLY RELIABLE

Before being accepted for publication, articles are submitted by the journal's editor to a peer review — a critique by other doctors and scientists who have expert knowledge in the subject of the paper. To ensure that the comments of these referees are freely and objectively given, their names are not revealed to the author of the article. The referees' responsibility is to verify the study's significance and its validity. Does it represent a contribution to medical science? Does it carry sufficient data to scientifically support its conclusions?

The peer review process attempts to ensure that a study meets the stringent requirements of scientific inquiry. Despite these high standards, journal articles are not perfect documents. Even though they deal in facts, those facts are sometimes open to interpretation. This is where you'll have to make decisions on your own.

If you feel overwhelmed when you first lay eyes on a journal article, remember that it has a specialized vocabulary and style. Once you sit down with a medical dictionary in hand, you'll become more comfortable — perhaps even engaged — with your new experience. Don't expect to understand everything, especially with one pass. As in a detective story, the clues are there if you dig for them. Keep in mind the points that follow in this chapter, and soon you will be able to glean exactly what you require from this specialized kind of literature.

THE STRUCTURE OF A MEDICAL JOURNAL ARTICLE

Medical journal articles (except for review articles, discussed below and in chapter 6) are subdivided into sections, typically in the following order:

Title

Journal article titles are intended to convey in as few words as possible what an article is about. Their precision is an asset but can occasionally be misleading. One individual recalls how he nearly ignored an article whose title described how a drug led to remissions of cancer in a "minority" of patients. The minority proved to be between 30 and 40 percent, far better odds than other alternatives offered. Usually, however, the titles of articles enable you to tell at a glance whether to read further.

Abstract

This serves as a brief summary of the essential details, such as why and how the study was conducted, what were its results, and what those results demonstrate. It appears at the top of the first page, usually in boldface type, to set it apart from the main body of the paper.

Abstracts enable you to decide whether you wish to read the whole article and, assuming that you do, to fix its main points in your mind. An experienced researcher offers one caution: the full text of an article may mention relevant exceptions to the article's main conclusion, and these exceptions may not be mentioned in the abstract.

Introduction

This describes a particular problem in the treatment of disease, introduces the present study, and tells why it may offer a solution (or partial solution) to that problem. Overall, it summarizes the main purpose of the study.

Methods

This section outlines what was studied, what was done (the surgical procedure, the administration of medications, and so forth), and how the data were measured (recurrence of disease, follow-up tests, and so forth).

Results

This section explains and elaborates upon the findings of the investigation.

Discussion, Summary, or Conclusions

This restates the main findings of the study and suggests how they may be used. In some cases, such a summary is presented at the end of the results section.

References

This section lists sources for information the author has borrowed. The number in front of each source corresponds to a superscript or number enclosed in a bracket or parentheses that appears in the text following the borrowed information. The references section appears at the end of the article. Note: *Review articles* list two or three times as many references as other studies, since they are a summary of information contained in numerous *other* articles.

Author Information

The main, or primary, author of an article is most often the first author listed, and this person is the one to contact if you have questions. The address of his or her institution is usually located in fine print on the first page at the bottom of the left-hand column. This is generally the same address as the one for reprint requests.

HOW SUZANNE LEARNED

Recall from the preface to this book that a doctor told Suzanne there was as much as a 25 percent chance that her mother's operation might prove fatal. The liver, he had explained, is full of veins and arteries that can bleed extensively; sometimes the bleeding can't be controlled. Because of this, many surgeons prefer removing an entire segment of the liver — one that is clearly bounded by a few main blood vessels — even if only a relatively small portion of that organ contains tumor. When there are multiple tumors, or tumors not confined to one of the two lobes into which the liver is divided, this method may not be feasible, because too much of the organ will have to be removed. The doctor, in fact, cautioned that he would not perform surgery at all if the tumor involved both lobes of the liver.

Suzanne found this prospect unacceptable. Rejecting the idea that her mother might undergo complex, dangerous surgery and end up not having her tumor removed, Suzanne (with her husband's help) began searching for medical journal articles that might present better prospects. Her intention was to discover (a) if the risk of surgery could be reduced, and (b) if there were surgeons who would operate no matter where the tumor was located.

Suzanne followed the method of searching for an article in *Index Medicus* and found Minton's paper, "Results of Surgical Excision of One to 13 Hepatic Metastases in 98 Consecutive Patients." Since the search method described in the previous chapter also helps reveal what the title of an article means, she knew that "hepatic" refers to the liver; "excision" stands for "cutting out of"; and "metastases" in cancer refers to the appearance of it in a part of the body remote from its first location.

What the Abstract Tells

The phrase "One to 13 Hepatic Metastases" in the title provided Suzanne with a flicker of hope that the author (a surgeon) had the ability to remove very small sections of the liver, as opposed to an entire lobe. It seemed a strong possibility, but she couldn't be sure just from the title. The abstract would be a good place to find out.

The abstract read:

Metastatic carcinoma to the liver is generally considered to be associated with a poor prognosis, with five-year survival of only 20% to 30% after resection of solitary lesions. Ninety-eight consecutive patients underwent the surgical removal of one to 13 metastatic lesions from the liver. A rising carcinoembryonic antigen level was considered an indication for reexploration. All gross tumor was removed in every patient; 66 had more than one metastasis . . . The procedure appears to be a safe and, in some patients, beneficial

surgical technique for the removal of multiple hepatic
metastases.

As formidable as these words sound, they can be broken down
into understandable sentences — each one conveying significant
information.

The abstract begins with the general statement, "Metastatic
carcinoma to the liver is generally considered to be associated with
a poor prognosis." In ordinary language, this means that when
cancer spreads to the liver, the outlook for the patient is not good.

Most scientific and medical journal articles (and abstracts) begin this way: they describe the overall expectations for a medical
situation at present and indicate whether the study in hand suggests the chance of an improved expectation.

The sentence beginning, "Ninety-eight consecutive patients"
announces the description of Minton's study. It notes that he used
the records of 98 patients in uninterrupted order, not skipping
any. If, for example, he had left out information on a patient who
died on the operating table or who had multiple, inoperable tumors, that would have changed his conclusions (and Suzanne's basis for optimism) significantly.

The sentence that follows, "A rising carcinoembryonic antigen
level," was not important to Suzanne at this point. She simply
noted that her mother's diagnosis, too, had been based in part on
the results of a carcinoembryonic antigen (CEA) test.

But the subsequent words — "All gross tumor was removed in
every patient; 66 had more than one metastasis" — brought welcome news. They meant that in Minton's group of 98 patients, he
was able to remove any and all known tumors on the liver.
(Suzanne reasoned that "gross tumor" must mean large enough to
be detectable.) Obviously, then, he hadn't removed the entire lobe
or segment of a liver, but a much smaller portion of tissue. The
methods section would yield more detail.

Suzanne was encouraged by the summarizing sentence, in
which Minton notes that the procedure "appears to be safe." But
to learn exactly what that meant she would have to find specific
references to mortality rates in the summary section of the text.
When she looked there, she read: "During the past seven years, 98

patients with one or more hepatic metastases (one to 13) have been operated on and all detectable metastatic tumor was removed, with acceptably low blood loss, no mortality, and low morbidity." Suzanne had found what she was looking for — and more. Minton had performed 98 operations over a seven-year period with minimal blood loss, few complications (morbidity), and *no* deaths.

For detail, she turned to the results section. There the author presented the figure for average amount of blood loss, after which appeared the following sentence: "No blood transfusions were given during the last 50 operations." This meant that blood loss — the great danger of liver surgery — had not even been a medical problem with the last 50 patients in the study. Suzanne could draw an important inference about Minton's capabilities as a surgeon: that he had honed his skills to an exceptionally high level. This was the sort of doctor she might well want for her mother.

In the methods section, Suzanne also found out exactly how Minton performed his surgery (with an electrocautery knife that seals a wound by burning and creating scar tissue) and minimized blood loss (metal clips placed at vessels, and finger counterpressure at the large vessels).

Encouraging data reflecting the number of years patients in the studied group survived after surgery emerged in the results section. There Suzanne read that 90 of the 98 patients were alive at the end of one year, 71 survived up to two years, 23 up to three years, and so forth. Four had survived beyond five years. These percentages were far better than the ones presented by the surgeons Suzanne's mother had consulted. When she was first diagnosed with recurrent cancer, she had not been expected to live more than eighteen months, and here were some of Minton's patients living three — even five — years. Perhaps, Suzanne thought, *someone* knows a way to give my mother a fighting chance.

Not all the information contained in Minton's article turned out to be relevant to Suzanne's search. As she scanned the results section, for example, she noticed a lengthy description of the sizes and shapes of the various excised tumors. This information had no bearing on her immediate concerns, although it was probably important to other surgeons, so she never bothered to give it detailed attention. You may find more data in a journal article than you require. Be judicious in your reading. Review the entire study, but save your energy for the sections that are pertinent to your needs.

References

As we've already noted, medical journal articles are often valuable not only for the contents of their text but for providing references to *other* articles that may be of help.

To illustrate, let us imagine that Suzanne had wished to learn in fuller detail about what might happen if her mother decided *not* to have surgery. Minton alluded to such cases in his introductory remarks: "The median survival of untreated patients with hepatic metastases ranges from 3.1 to nine months.[1]" The superscript number led Suzanne to the first citation in the reference section. There, Minton gave credit to his source: "1. Jaffe BM, Donegan WL, Watson F et al: Factors influencing survival in patients with untreated hepatic metastases. *Surg Gynecol Obstet* 1968;127:1–11." This citation provides all the publishing information — authors, title, journal title, date, volume, and page — necessary to locate the article. Suzanne could have learned all she needed to know about the survival rates of different classes of patients with untreated liver metastases from that study.

Reference notes, then, are an important means of finding more studies on a subject. Always check the references section. An important article might turn up, one that you could have missed in your original search simply because the key words were a bit different than those you used, or because you hadn't thought of that particular aspect of the subject.

Suzanne took her mother to Columbus, Ohio, where Dr. Minton operated. During surgery, he discovered that the tumor was located at the junction of the liver where the two lobes meet. Since his method allowed him to remove a tumor even when both lobes were involved, he excised the entire cancerous lesion. Suzanne's mother (seventy-five years old at the time) lost only about one-quarter of a cup of blood and withstood the surgery extremely well. Had the first surgeon operated, he would not have excised the tumor, since it involved both lobes of the liver. And, as the statistic cited above made all too clear, without surgical removal, her mother could not be expected to live out the year. As noted in the preface, Suzanne's mother not only survived her surgery, but lived a full life with her malignancy controlled. Her death, four years later, was not due to her cancer.

LARGE CASE STUDY GROUPS AND CLINICAL TRIALS

The article that Suzanne read, "Results of Surgical Excision," is an example of a case report, a study that reports on findings within a relatively small population. From such a paper you'd be most apt to learn about *new* or innovative techniques and treatments practiced on a fairly small scale and not widely known. However, it should be remembered that such studies do not use control groups (which provide comparison data on those patients receiving "standard" treatment).

For some kinds of searches you'll require strong statistical evidence and comprehensive data, available only from large, randomized, controlled, double-blind studies, which track hundreds of patients. If you needed to find comparison material on two well-known treatments, for instance, you would want to see such a study. The medical-scientific community (especially the providers of large grants, such as the National Institutes of Health, NIH) supports such larger studies, frequently after smaller ones have paved the way.

Large-group studies can provide an abundance of information. Because they report on hundreds or thousands of cases, they are more conclusive than smaller studies. In addition, they are *prospective*, meaning that they are carefully planned to yield statistically valid information. (Case studies, such as those reported in Dr. Minton's paper, are generally *retrospective* and look at data from the past.)

If you're looking for *comparative detail* — trying to contrast the benefits and risks of two or more therapies, for example — clinical trials will provide you with the most substantial information available.

The story of Bob Long, a fifty-five-year-old mathematician who lives near Boston, illustrates how useful such an article can be.

During a routine physical examination, the doctor heard an irregular sound in one of Bob's carotid arteries. These large arteries (one on each side of the neck) fork near the head to form inner and outer branches that deliver blood to the brain.

The sound (called "bruit" — the French word for "noise") indicated that one or both branches of the carotid artery on Bob's right side were abnormally narrow. The doctor explained that this condition, known as *stenosis*, is caused by hardened fatty deposits and can lead to the formation of blood clots. The clots can break off and migrate to the brain, causing stroke.

Sometimes stenosis will produce warning symptoms — visual irregularities or numbness, for instance — caused by tiny clots. The doctor asked if Bob had experienced any such warnings, but he hadn't. This meant that his stenosis was *asymptomatic* — without symptoms. Only the doctor's detection of the bruit revealed the condition — one that could lead to a large clot and catastrophic stroke without an earlier signal.

The doctor (a general physician) referred Bob to a neurologist. An ultrasound test, which applies an imaging technique using sound waves, confirmed the fatty deposits in Bob's carotid artery and indicated a blockage in the range of 75 to 95 percent. The neurologist told Bob he might be a candidate for a *carotid endarterectomy*, surgery to remove the artery blockage. This procedure, the doctor told him, is recommended when the patient's artery is 70 percent or more obstructed. To know whether he required an operation, Bob needed a test called an angiogram to obtain an even more accurate measurement of the stenosis than the ultrasound test had provided. (An angiograph uses X-rays with dye injected directly into the diseased vessel for visual contrast.)

The results of Bob's angiogram revealed a 60 to 70 percent stenosis, making him a borderline case, in which the consequences of opting for or against surgery were not distinct. The decision, according to the doctor, would be up to Bob.

"I don't know how to decide," Bob told his brother John. John offered to help by performing a MEDLINE search (as described in chapters 10 and 11) at the university where he worked.

The search located an article in the *New England Journal of Medicine:* "Beneficial Effect of Carotid Endarterectomy in Symptomatic Patients with High-Grade Carotid Stenosis." The authors were described as North American Symptomatic Carotid Endarterectomy Trial (NASCET) Collaborators. (Henceforth, the article will be referred to as "NASCET trial.") The word "trial" signified to John that this was a big study with ample data. The abstract bore this out: "We conducted a randomized trial at 50 clinical centers . . . We report here the results in [the] 659 patients. . . ."

Satisfied that he had found the right *kind* of study (one with a large sample population), John turned his attention to the article.

This is part of the abstract John read:

> *Background.* Without strong evidence of benefit, the use of carotid endarterectomy for prophylaxis against stroke rose dramatically until the mid 1980s, then declined. Our investigation sought to determine whether carotid endarterectomy reduces the risk of stroke among patients with a recent adverse cerebrovascular event and ipsilateral carotid stenosis.

The abstract as a whole implies that doctors were not sure whether endarterectomy was justified as a preventive measure against stroke. The purpose of this study had been to answer that question.

After checking for some definitions in a medical dictionary, John understood the words in lay terms to mean that the study was restricted to patients who had experienced symptoms of their stenosis. ("Ipsilateral" means "on the same side" and indicates that the "event" is caused by the stenosis because it involves the same side). The patients in the study had experienced adverse cerebrovascular (blood vessels relating to the brain) events and other overt symptoms, probably the visual disturbance or numbness Bob's doctor had asked him about.

Although Bob and the group studied shared one characteristic — significant stenosis — the group was not completely representative of Bob's case. Recall that he was "asymptomatic" and had not as yet suffered an "adverse cerebrovascular event." Even though the study did not match his brother's case exactly, John's attention was drawn by the conclusions in the abstract: "Carotid endarterectomy is highly beneficial to . . . [symptomatic] . . . patients with high-grade stenosis (70 to 99 percent) of the internal carotid artery." Since surgery was so clearly beneficial to symptomatic patients, the study might also be relevant to those, like his brother, who were asymptomatic. To learn more, he turned to the main text and the "methods" section.

RESEARCH METHODS AND RANDOMIZATION

In the methods section John learned that the designers of the study restricted participation to high-quality medical centers with top-notch surgical teams: "Each center had a rate of less than 6 percent for stroke and death occurring within 30 days of operation for at least 50 consecutive carotid endarterectomies performed within the previous 24 months. . . ."

John would stress this information to his brother. If Bob did select surgery, he would have to remember that the journal article's conclusions applied *only* to exceptionally good medical centers where there had been, over a two-year period, an unbroken succession of at least fifty endarterectomies with a low rate (less than 6 percent) of death or complications from surgery.

This conclusion was underscored in the discussion section:

We caution readers not to apply our conclusions too broadly. First, the study surgeons were selected only after audits of their endarterectomy results by our surgical committee confirmed a high level of expertise. If comparable expertise and quality control are not achieved in the widespread implementation of these results and the perioperative [around the time of surgery] risk of major stroke and death exceeds the 2.1 percent reported here, the benefit of endarterectomy will diminish. If the rate of major complications approaches 10 percent, the benefit will vanish entirely.

This demonstrated that, if Bob selected surgery, he should look for a surgical team with a low rate of complications. If a surgical team's rate of complications approached 10 percent, there would be a greater danger of stroke than there would be from not having the surgery at all.

To produce significant data, scientists and doctors try to ensure that the process of selecting patients who take part in a study does not in itself influence the outcome. The best way to achieve neutrality is through randomization. Researchers use random numbers generated by [a] computer to assign patients to a group (surgery or nonsurgery, for example). This was the selection procedure used in the NASCET trial. John learned of it in the methods section: "patients were randomly assigned to receive either medical care alone or medical care plus surgery, according to a computer-generated randomization schedule." This meant that patients entering the study had an equal chance of being placed by the computer in either the surgical or nonsurgical group. Further on in the methods section, John discovered a surprising assertion:

> On February 1, 1991, the trial's preplanned rule for stopping randomization was invoked because of evidence of treatment efficacy [in those] who underwent carotid endarterectomy. On February 21, the monitoring and executive committees agreed that randomization of patients . . . should be stopped. . . .

All trials require a board of experts to monitor data and review the progress of the study. In this case, the board ordered that randomization be stopped because the incoming data unequivocally demonstrated the beneficial results of surgery. It would have been unethical not to make these advantageous results available to all participants in the study. For John, this decision by the monitoring board was eloquent testimony to the effectiveness of surgery.

INTERPRETING ARTICLES AND EDITORIALS

The NASCET trial article John studied was nine pages long, and complex. He concentrated on getting the information he needed and avoided material that went into great detail about methods and statistical formulations. In the results section, he found key information: there was a 26 percent risk of stroke in the 331 patients receiving aspirin only compared to a 9 percent risk of stroke in the 328 patients also receiving surgery. This, then, began to look to John like compelling evidence for his brother to undergo surgery, even though the groups studied did not exactly parallel his medical history. But he still wasn't certain. Bob, after all, was healthy now, and his stenosis was at the low end of high risk.

Fortunately, John had found one more article, although it wasn't a study. Published in the same issue as the *New England Journal of Medicine* article on the NASCET trial (August 15, 1991) was an editorial commenting on its significance. As is often the case when a major study comes out, the journal in which it appears had issued an accompanying editorial (discussed below).

An editorial like this is worth looking for when you search for medical articles; it offers several advantages. One is its narrative style, which is much friendlier and easier to follow than the scientific format. Often, too, the editor discusses other studies (ones you may well not have researched) to draw comparisons or conclusions. Finally, it is often not easy to interpret journal articles or derive ready conclusions from them. An advantage of editorials, then, is that they are generally written by highly qualified physicians and provide an independent and competent evaluation of the data. Such editorials, as John discovered, are an excellent added resource.

EVALUATING WHAT YOU READ IN PERSONAL TERMS

John read the entire editorial, entitled "Carotid Endarterectomy — Specific Therapy Based on Pathophysiology." Its comments on the NASCET trial study clarified some issues. For example, he was able to find a specific reference to borderline cases that he had somehow missed in the first paper: "the efficacy of the procedure was clear even in patients with lesions causing only 70 percent stenosis." This meant that Bob could very possibly benefit from surgery, even though he wasn't far up in the highest-risk group.

John also found a discussion of patients who, like his brother, had experienced no symptoms:

> In [asymptomatic] cases the recommended strategy has been to control the risk factors for atherosclerosis — that is, hypertension, hypercholesterolemia, and smoking. A low dose of aspirin may be a useful precaution. However, embolism from a high-grade, hemodynamically important stenotic lesion is the most common cause of cerebral symptoms resulting from that lesion. The first symptom may not be simply a transient neurologic deficit or a minor stroke but instead a severe stroke.

This meant that Bob might try to treat his condition by following certain precautions, such as reducing high blood pressure and cholesterol. However, John also read in the editorial, "there has been no reliable medical therapy to reduce the extent of an atherosclerotic lesion once it has formed. . . ." That is, without surgery, the hardened fatty deposit (atherosclerotic lesion) in Bob's carotid artery would remain or become worse. Surgery could be deferred until Bob became symptomatic, but there was a real possibility that his first symptom could be a devastating stroke.

Bob, after considering all the factors, decided to choose surgery. He was fairly young and in good physical shape. If he delayed surgery, he might wind up being operated on when he was weakened by age, had additional medical problems, and probably a progression of his disease. He knew, too, as John had explained, that hand-in-hand with his decision for surgery went the necessity of selecting a high-quality hospital and medical team.

With the help of the articles his brother found, and then conferring with a vascular surgeon, Bob was able to make a well-thought-out, reasoned medical decision. His operation was successful, and he experienced no complications. The surgery, incidentally, revealed a 70 to 75 percent stenosis, which meant that he had been in a higher-risk group than he had realized.

Since the NASCET trial, a new large study has been completed that verifies the benefit of surgery for asymptomatic patients with 70 percent or greater stenosis.

≈

You don't have to be a doctor to understand the main points of journal articles. But keep a medical dictionary close at hand and remember to focus only on what you need to learn from the study. Use its organization to help you find information.

In a series of articles published for physicians by the *Journal of the American Medical Association* in 1993 and 1994 ("Users' Guides to the Medical Literature"), a group of experts outline principles for evaluating the research design and quality of data on which medical journal articles are based. Highlights from these principles offer a guide for evaluating many of the articles you may study:

• In studies comparing treatments, was the assignment of patients to treatments randomized, thereby eliminating the possibility of bias in assigning patients to one treatment group or another?
• Were all patients who entered the study accounted for, so that those patients who did not complete the study did not bias the study's conclusion?
• Were patients, clinicians, and study personnel "blind" to treatment, thus preventing bias in patient behavior or clinical treatment?
• Was the study follow-up of sufficient duration to predict long-term prognosis?
• Was the treatment effect more than a minor improvement, and did it affect final outcome?
• Were all important outcomes considered? For example, did a reported reduction in tumor size extend life expectancy?
• Are the treatment benefits worth the potential harm and costs?

With regard to specific criteria relative to your own needs:

- Does the study reported here relate directly to your medical problem?
- If not, does it still yield valuable information?
- Is there an accompanying editorial that would help you interpret and evaluate the study?
- Does the article reveal any treatment alternatives not previously considered?
- Do the references disclose any other studies that may be of interest?
- Does the author or his institution specialize in the treatment of this condition?
- Would it help you to contact the author directly for more information?
- Have you tailored your reading to concentrate on the sections of the article that are specifically relevant to your medical history?

If reading a medical journal article seems difficult, remember that neither Suzanne nor John had medical training. Yet by using the methods described in this chapter, they were able to gather important information from journal articles — information that allowed them to help people they loved to survive life-threatening illnesses.

8.

Information from Organizations

GAYLE ALLISON LEARNED about alternatives to conventional acoustic neuroma surgery from a national organization, the Acoustic Neuroma Association. Similarly, Gary Schine's contacts with the Leukemia Society of America set him on the way to the discovery of a successful treatment — one he had not heard about from his doctor.

Although you may not get that kind of direct and dramatic help from an organization that concerns itself with your medical problem, you should take full advantage of the resources of patient-oriented organizations and groups. They are important sources of information about treatment options and can save you substantial amounts of time, not only in locating medical information but in interpreting it and applying it to your individual situation. Because the information they collect relates to a specific subject, it is often more accessible than general medical collections and more likely to be focused on your needs.

Patient-oriented organizations can help you in other ways. Their members typically include individuals who have had, or may still have, medical problems like your own. They can provide

what one organization executive calls "experiential" information —
for example, what to expect at a hospital, how you're likely to
feel after taking a particular kind of medication, where to buy
products that can make your recovery easier. Needless to add, they
can also be an invaluable source of moral support and encouragement at a time when you may need that badly. Moreover, many organizations perform advocacy work on behalf of patients and their
families. This function may not interest you while your energies
are absorbed in your own search for the best treatment. Later on,
it may.

There are, of course, thousands of national, regional, state,
and local organizations working in health-related fields — far
too many even to list here, much less to describe. This chapter
briefly discusses only six of them. They include four national organizations: the National Kidney Cancer Association (NKCA),
the National Marrow Donor Program (NMDP), Patient Advocates for Advanced Cancer Treatments (PAACT), and the National Organization for Rare Disorders (NORD). A fifth group,
the Community Breast Health Project, is a community-based
organization of a kind that you should know about, whether or
not anything like it exists in your geographical area. Finally, a
sixth group, the People's Medical Society, is included for its role
in providing consumer information on the systemic aspects of
health care — for example, on hospitals, medical records, and
patients' rights.

These organizations, although a tiny fraction of the total, illustrate some of the different roles groups play and should suffice to
suggest how you can benefit from what groups have to offer.

NATIONAL KIDNEY CANCER ASSOCIATION

In the span of only a few years, the National Kidney Cancer Association (NKCA), founded in 1990, has acquired a reputation as an
unusually strong patient organization. Eugene Schonfeld, Ph.D.,
the president and chief executive officer of NKCA and himself a
kidney cancer patient, has helped establish a group that is guided
by the same principles espoused in this book: patients should be

completely informed about their disease and its treatment, especially newer options.

To that end, the NKCA offers a wide array of services — all with the goal of providing the means for kidney cancer patients to learn about and take advantage of the latest scientific advances in the treatment of their disease.

Patients calling the NKCA headquarters in Evanston, Illinois, will hear a human voice and receive immediate information about any aspects of kidney cancer, including well-written, well-documented literature. If they want the name of a physician, the NKCA can refer them to a qualified specialist. (The NKCA's medical advisory board is also available to consult with a patient's physician.)

For patients wanting to explore the scientific literature with help from the NKCA, including information from the National Cancer Institute about clinical trials, the association makes it available through its computer bulletin board system, with which patients can connect (by a toll-free number) either from home or a public library. The association can also put patients in touch with scientists working on specific projects in the field of kidney cancer.

The list of NKCA activities includes an annual convention of patients and expert doctors in the field of kidney cancer brought together to discuss the newest therapies for the disease, insurance and legal assistance, public policy and advocacy programs to promote the approval of new drugs by the Food and Drug Administration (FDA), and direct support of kidney cancer research.

NATIONAL MARROW DONOR PROGRAM

The primary function of the National Marrow Donor Program (NMDP) is to help patients in need of a bone marrow transplant from an unrelated (nonfamily) donor find an acceptable match. NMDP keeps a computerized registry of information on the tissue types of approximately one million volunteer donors throughout the United States (and foreign registries when requested) who are willing to share their marrow if called upon. As such, the

NMDP, a congressionally authorized program, already provides a lifesaving service to patients with aplastic anemia, acute and chronic leukemia, some lymphomas, some solid tumor cancers, and other diseases, whose best (or only) hope is to receive a bone marrow transplant.

This unique organization also provides direct services to patients who contact it for information. People who have just been told by their doctors that they may need a bone marrow transplant often find themselves in a kind of limbo during the sometimes long process of finding a match. The patient's specialist (probably a medical oncologist or hematologist) is rarely directly involved in the search for a match, and the specialist and the team who will perform the transplant must wait until an appropriate donor is found. In the meantime, the patient may have many questions his or her doctor cannot answer.

For such patients, the NMDP performs an extraordinarily helpful service. Callers to the NMDP toll-free number (answered by a human being) are promptly put in touch with a patient advocate who will answer questions about any phase of the bone marrow transplant process, from how long finding a match may take to what the procedure will entail. In addition, NMDP staff members conduct medical literature searches for patients requesting them. And patients with problems relating to their health insurance receive help from staff members with expert knowledge in insurance coverage for bone marrow transplants.

The jewel of NMDP's information program is a publication called the *Transplant Center Access Directory*. Patients can request a copy of this spiral-bound annual compendium, which lists all the accredited, NMDP-participating transplant centers with significant information about each one. It includes a general description of the institution, survival and remission rates, the types of diseases the institution will treat with a marrow transplant, its criteria for tissue match and age of patient, contact information for the referring doctor, and the name of the program coordinator. Since the success of a bone marrow transplant, as with many other procedures, depends a great deal upon the experience of the physicians and the record of the institution where it's performed, the information in the access directory is invaluable.

PATIENT ADVOCATES FOR ADVANCED CANCER TREATMENTS

Despite a name that suggests a broad mission, Patient Advocates for Advanced Cancer Treatments (PAACT) concentrates its educational and other efforts entirely on prostate cancer, the second largest cause of cancer death among American males.

PAACT publishes a large body of printed materials on prostate cancer, including a 67-page booklet that describes different stages of prostate cancer and treatment options for each stage — usually several of them. For example, *seven* treatment options are discussed for Stage B tumors, meaning tumors that have reached a readily detectable size but are not judged likely to have spread beyond the prostate gland itself. There's also a brief, clear description of tests for prostate cancer and how to interpret them. Much of the language of the booklet appears to have been excerpted directly from medical journal articles, although citations are generally lacking.

PAACT offers a model folder entitled "My Personal Medical Record," designed to facilitate a patient's records management and note-taking during physician conferences. PAACT also publishes a bimonthly newsletter, *Cancer Communication*, containing references to recent technical literature and opinion pieces from patients. PAACT insists that the current "gold standard" treatments for prostate cancer (complete surgical removal of the prostate gland and radiation therapy) have not been demonstrated to be superior to other treatments. The organization's outspoken insistence that prostate cancer patients should be informed of *all* mainstream medical options has drawn fire from some physicians.

NATIONAL ORGANIZATION FOR RARE DISORDERS

The National Organization for Rare Disorders (NORD) is a non-profit group devoted to dissemination of information on so-called "orphan diseases." It has individual members, but it is also a federation of over 135 nonprofit health-related organizations, each focusing on one or more rare diseases. NORD defines a rare disease as one affecting fewer than 200,000 Americans — that is, fewer than one person per thousand. Some of the disorders with which NORD deals are considerably rarer than that, and many physicians see them too seldom for easy diagnosis. In fact, the NORD newsletter, *Orphan Disease Update*, which is published three times a year, asserts that one out of three individuals with a rare disease does not receive a correct diagnosis for up to five years.

Over seventy-five thousand people contact NORD directly each year, and more than two hundred thousand access its Rare Disease Databases, available on CompuServe and elsewhere. The organization operates a medication assistance program to help financially needy individuals to receive expensive drugs. NORD also publishes the *Physicians' Guide to Rare Diseases.*

The NORD files include articles on approximately one thousand diseases. Some of these diseases are not rare, but NORD includes them because it gets numerous requests for information on them. If you indicate the disorder that concerns you, the NORD research staff will provide you with a report on the disease. The first report is free, and subsequent ones are four dollars.

COMMUNITY BREAST HEALTH PROJECT

The Community Breast Health Project (CBHP), Palo Alto, California, was founded in 1993 by a surgeon and one of her breast cancer patients, who together decided that women with breast cancer needed more guidance and support than most were receiving from their physicians. Several hundred women joined in brainstorming sessions on the group's potential roles. All agreed on the need for more information, both clinical and experiential. This organization is grassroots, patient-centered, and all its services are free.

Visitors to the CBHP office will find binders crammed with information about medical issues such as breast cancer treatments, screening techniques, and research. They'll also find tips on practical matters like sources for low-cost screening mammography, psychological support for family members, and where to buy wigs (which may be needed during chemotherapy).

The organization operates a hotline, staffed by volunteers. Callers receive information and, if needed, help in finding a "buddy" — a person who has had a similar breast cancer prognosis and/or treatment. "Buddies" provide moral support and perhaps more tangible assistance, such as accompanying patients on visits to a physician to help with questions, note-taking, or use of a tape recorder. Anyone with complex needs is referred to more extensive support programs.

The CBHP also sponsors a speaker series. The speakers are mainly health professionals but have also included attorneys and insurance experts. One evening each week, CBHP sponsors a "drop-in" open house where any patient, family member, or friend can speak with a physician about breast cancer and listen to what other patients or professionals have to say. Volunteers are available to assist patients in online searches of medical databases. Finally, CBHP offers volunteer opportunities for patients as well as health care providers, believing that patients regain a sense of self-worth and emotional strength from helping others.

The CBHP is creating its own online database that patients with personal computers can search from their homes. To deal with the problems of treatment choice, CBHP is also developing ways to help patients understand the options they have in a battle with cancer, from diagnosis through primary treatment and supplemental therapies.

Local groups that perform as many functions as CBHP are, of course, rare. Nevertheless, you should make efforts to find out what exists in your area, either by contacting a national organization or local health groups.

PEOPLE'S MEDICAL SOCIETY

The People's Medical Society differs from the other groups listed here in that it is *not* a direct source of information on specific diseases, except through the sale of books on common disorders like arthritis, diabetes, allergies, and prostate cancer. It is, however, one of the largest and most aggressive health care consumer groups in the nation. Its overall focus is consumer education.

Founded in 1982 by the late Robert Rodale, publisher of *Prevention* magazine, the People's Medical Society is a membership organization. Members receive a monthly newsletter and discounts on its publications. The People's Medical Society takes an aggressive patients'-rights stance. *U.S. News & World Report* once referred to its president, Charles B. Inlander, as the "Ralph Nader of health care." The organization advocates broad changes in the American health care delivery system, including elimination of "pre-existing condition" exclusions from insurance policies and public access to a practitioner data bank providing information on aspects of physicians' performance. These and other positions suffice to make many doctors wary of the group.

Getting the best medical care is not merely a question of which drugs you take or which therapies you choose. Whatever your reaction to the legal and political positions taken by the People's Medical Society, you may benefit from its book list, which includes many books published by the society and several by other publishers. One of its most popular titles, *Take This Book to the Hospital with You*, despite its somewhat adversarial tone, is a useful reminder of how to avoid problems that may be associated with hospitalization.

HOW PATIENT ORGANIZATIONS DIFFER

All of the six patient-centered groups described above perform several functions. You may or may not find an organization for your own purposes that offers you as much as several of these do. Some groups provide a few pamphlets that give you a simply worded summary of the kind of information that you will find in the books described in chapter 5, accompanied by a bland assurance that your friendly physician will be glad to answer any additional questions you may have.

Unfortunately, there's no way to know in advance which organizations emphasize hard data, which emphasize moral support, and which may have a bias toward their own special agenda. You can, however, tell a lot about a group's objectivity by the tone of its literature. Be cautious of organizations pushing one treatment option to the near-exclusion of all others, whether that option is an alternative therapy like bee pollen or something well within the medical mainstream. Even if the option happened to be the best treatment available for most people at the time the group's focus was set, it may not be the best treatment for *you* now. This could be true for either of two reasons: (a) the state of the art has changed faster than the group's thinking or (b) something about your own situation makes the group's recommended treatment inappropriate.

In short, you must be prepared to evaluate the information you receive from patient-oriented groups by the same standards you would apply to that from any other source: relevance, evidence of scientific authority, and recency. Just as doctors have difficulty in keeping up with recent medical developments, so do self-help groups. Moreover, individuals in a patient-oriented group may not be trained in scientific or medical evaluation. Their views are almost inevitably colored by the positive and negative aspects of their prior experiences with their own physicians.

LOCATING GROUPS THAT CAN HELP

The easiest way to locate patient-centered organizations (whose members may include physicians and other health-care professionals) is to contact the American Self-Help Clearinghouse, Saint Clare's-Riverside Medical Center, Denville, NJ 07834, (201) 625-7101. The clearinghouse publishes *The Self-Help Sourcebook: Finding and Forming Mutual Aid Self-Help Groups*, now in its fifth edition. It is available for ten dollars and contains the names, addresses, phone numbers, and a short description of more than eight hundred organizations. A few names are likely to sound familiar: for example, the Arthritis Foundation and the United Cerebral Palsy Associations. Many others provide a way of connecting people with relatively rare disorders or special problems that may be associated with more than one disorder: for example, the Ankylosing Spondylitis Association, the Beckwith-Wiedemann Support Network, the National Chronic Pain Outreach Association, and the International Ventilator User Network. The organizations listed in the *Sourcebook* may perform any or all of three functions: emotional support, education, and political advocacy.

"Many people seek out these groups," says Edward J. Madara, executive director of the American Self-Help Clearinghouse, "just to talk with someone who truly understands what it's like because they've been there. I was on the phone recently talking with a woman who was interested in forming a group for parents of children with what's called cyclic vomiting syndrome. There's no known cure, but they'll be coming together to share what they've done in coping."

Experiential education occurs when people pool their coping skills and the practical information they've gathered on how to deal with problems they have in common. Newsletters published by self-help organizations often contain highly specific suggestions on such matters as dealing with doctors unfamiliar with certain problems, purchasing and using medical products and equipment, organizing a home or workplace around disabilities, and explaining unusual symptoms to strangers.

Many of the listed groups provide pamphlets, citations, and copies of medical journal articles dealing with the conditions that affect their members. The amount of such material will range from minuscule to extensive, depending on the organization's resources. Similarly, some groups are able to provide material without charge; others will charge for some items or ask for contributions.

WHAT IF NO SELF-HELP GROUP EXISTS FOR YOU?

"Some of the people who call us looking for help," says Madara, "wind up creating their own organizations." He adds that many of the groups listed in the guide published by the Self-Help Clearinghouse "operate out of kitchen-table offices" and says that many national organizations began that way. "The National Multiple Sclerosis Society [which now has over seven hundred local chapters] was started by a woman whose brother had MS," he says. "The Huntington's Disease Society was started by the wife of the folk singer Woody Guthrie, who just pulled together some friends and families."

When you're actively searching for a treatment for yourself or someone you love, forming an organization may be the furthest thing from your mind. Nevertheless, you should be aware that the American Self-Help Clearinghouse can provide a limited amount of technical assistance on how to do that. If, of course, there's already a patient-support organization in existence somewhere that deals with your problem, you may be able to use it as a model for a local or regional group in your area.

Why would you want to do that?

Emotional support and altruism aside, Madara says that one answer is "respect." Organizations, even organizations without real budgets, are often able to attract physician-lecturers or other experts to meet with them.

The American Self-Help Clearinghouse itself evolved from a single New Jersey hospital's desire to identify patient-support groups within its own area. It became national almost without planning, simply in response to needs.

"There are these fabulous people out there," Madara says, "who just say, 'Other people shouldn't have to go through what I'm going through alone.' "

SEEING YOUR TREATMENT PROCESS AS A WHOLE

As a broad generalization, you can expect active members of patient-oriented groups to be at least as likely as the average physician in general practice to know the literature that pertains to their particular conditions. The best groups are governed by sophisticated individuals who have, or have had recently, the strongest possible incentive to keep abreast of promising developments or to get early warning of a treatment's potential dangers.

You should not, of course, regard what organizations provide as a *substitute* for consulting with a physician who knows your own condition well or for doing your own research. Almost without exception, however, the people who are active in patient-centered groups are eager to help you make the best medical decision you can. Perhaps even more important, they can add a new dimension to your thinking, helping you to see how particular treatment decisions fit into a long-term healing process. You are, after all, much more than your disease. You're an individual in your own right, and you have a family, friends, a job, and many other relationships. Your medical condition affects these relationships, and they in turn can enhance or inhibit your recovery. People who have "been there" can help you keep those relationships positive.

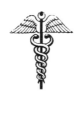

PART III

YOU CAN MASTER

ONLINE SEARCHING

Once you have a personal computer connected to your home telephone, you can roam the stacks of immense online libraries containing millions of published articles. You can also reach out for advice from medical specialists and support from individuals who know what you're going through because they've been there. Learning to search online databases and to find knowledgeable individuals eager to help is easier than people who haven't used computers realize. Commercial services are making computer-assisted telecommunications simpler and less expensive than ever. Even the once-mysterious Internet has become accessible to searchers with little computer experience.

9.

Computer Research
Fundamentals

THE YOUNG MAN in Lauren Langford's office wanted to talk to another man, a man who'd understand exactly what he was going through. That wasn't going to be easy; his illness was breast cancer.

Langford, a volunteer with the Community Breast Health Project (CBHP), located in Palo Alto, helps find "buddies" for breast cancer patients. Because breast cancer occurs in fewer than one in one hundred thousand males, the odds were very much against her finding another male with the disease anywhere in Palo Alto or any nearby area.

So Langford went online. She logged on to a discussion group on the Internet that focuses on breast cancer, one frequented by physicians and researchers. Almost immediately someone suggested a name. Unfortunately, it was the name of the man on whose behalf she was searching.

"I told you guys it was rare," she wrote back to the Internet group, "but I didn't think you'd have to match him up with himself."

That setback was temporary. She soon found the young man a "buddy" in New York, then another in Utah. Later, she was contacted by an organization that publicizes the needs of breast cancer patients by sponsoring benefit races in various cities around the country. She obtained a roster of male runners who listed themselves as breast cancer patients when signing up for those races. Now the young man who sought help from CBHP and his new friends seem to be on the way toward becoming the nucleus of a nationwide male breast cancer support group. These men's newfound ability to share both emotional support and information would simply not have been possible without access to a computer-based telecommunications network.

BRINGING THE WORLD OF MEDICINE INTO YOUR HOME

As you consider what computers can do for you, think first about how helpful it would be to have a huge medical library in your own home. Then consider how good it would be to know that you can, like the young man with breast cancer, reach out at any hour of the day or night and find help from people who've been through what you're going through — who understand your symptoms, your treatment's side effects, your frustrations, your fears. And while you're at it, imagine being coached on what to ask your own doctor by some of the top medical researchers in the country — none of whom ever sends you a bill.

Forget fantasy. You can in fact do all of this with a home computer. And this is true wherever you live — not just in major cities like New York and Los Angeles, but in places far from major population centers, like Ridgeview, North Dakota, and Pea Ridge, Arkansas.

Please don't dismiss the possibility of doing your own computer-assisted medical searches just because you may never have used a computer before. You can apply the principles of this book without a computer, but you'll find more current and more comprehensive information with one, not to mention the personal contacts with patients and physicians from all over the country.

This chapter and the four chapters that follow approach computer-assisted medical information searches from varying perspectives. *This chapter is nontechnical,* intended merely to give you a bird's-eye view of how you can use a personal computer as a medical research tool. For readers with no experience in computer-assisted telecommunications, it contains a very brief description of the equipment required. It also describes in a general way the variety of medical resources accessible by computer and how to make connections with these resources.

COMPUTER AND MODEM BASICS

If you're already familiar with the use of both computers and modems, you can skip this section. Read it if you have no experience with computers, or if you've used them only for tasks like word processing or spreadsheet calculations but not for telecommunications.

This and subsequent chapters often refer to *online* searches, *online* communications, and so on. *Online* means any activity that takes place over ordinary phone lines connecting two or more computers at widely separated locations. For example, an *online database* means a body of information stored in a remote "host" computer somewhere to which you (and your computer) connect. While you are actually connected, you are said to be *online*. Fees for access to information in a remote database, if determined by how long you are online, are called *online charges*. Obviously, the opposite of *online* is *offline*. To reduce online charges, do your planning and reading offline, insofar as possible.

The computer itself and any physical devices attached to it (printers, for example) are known as *hardware*. Other than the computer and a printer, the only hardware you'll need for doing computer-assisted searches to remote locations (online searches) is a *modem*. This device makes it possible for a computer to communicate with other computers via telephone lines. It converts data (text, numbers, even pictures) into electrical impulses that travel over telephone wires. When they reach their destination, another modem at the remote computer (known as the "host" computer if you're connecting to a database) converts them back into a form that can be recognized and acted upon by the host.

If you're adding a modem to a computer that doesn't have one, you can add either an "internal" or an "external" model. Their function is identical, and they both connect to your telephone with ordinary phone cables and jacks.

An external modem comes in a box about the size of a fat paperback book. It connects by one cable to your telephone and by another to a "serial port" in the back of your computer. (Verify, with the help of a knowledgeable friend if necessary, that your machine does have a serial port vacant.) The advantages of an external modem are that you don't have to open up the computer to install it and you can transfer it easily from one computer to another. The disadvantages are that it takes up space on a desk and it costs somewhat more than an internal modem.

An internal modem is simply a printed circuit board (called a "card") that goes inside your computer case. You can install one by pressing its bottom edge into an open slot on a board that holds other such cards. It'll be harder than changing a light bulb and easier than changing the oil in a car. (Just be sure to unplug the computer from its power source and to touch its metal case to discharge any static electricity from your clothing.)

If you're buying a new computer, get one with an internal modem already installed.

Modems differ in the speed with which they permit messages to be transmitted (measured in units called "bauds," such as 2400, 9600, or 14,400 baud). If you need to transfer large files from a remote computer to your own, the ability to do this at higher speeds can save a significant amount of time and money in telephone bills and other charges. A new modem will almost certainly be capable of sending and receiving at faster speeds than many of the remote computers to which you'll be connected. If you have an older modem that operates only at speeds of 1200 baud and below, you may want to upgrade it before doing much online searching.

Some areas lack local-call numbers for higher-speed modems, so you will sometimes find it economical to connect at a slower speed than your modem's maximum capacity. Note also that the speed of a given transaction can be no faster than that permitted by the slower of the two modems involved. For example, if your new modem will transmit and receive at 14,400 baud but the computer at the other end of the line from you can handle only 2400 baud, your modem will adjust to the slower speed, usually automatically.

If you're buying or upgrading a computer, you may want to consider the addition of a CD-ROM drive for between $100 and $300 and marketed as "multimedia." This equipment is *not* a necessity, but more and more medical resources are appearing in CD-ROM format, a technology that permits storage of immense amounts of data on a single disk. For new buyers, CD-ROM drives on home computers have moved from the "nice-to-have" to the "foolish-not-to-have" category.

In addition to hardware, you'll also need *software*, meaning programs that enable the computer to do what you want it to do. Software falls into two broad categories — "operating systems," which work in the background to enable the machine to work at all (rather like your autonomic nervous system, which controls basic bodily functions like heartbeat and respiration, without your having to think about it) and "applications," which enable the computer to do things like word processing, spreadsheets, and telecommunications. Programs like MS-DOS and Windows are examples of operating systems for IBM-compatible machines. Apple computers have built-in routines that perform the same basic functions.

Communications software handles the mechanics of making connections and managing the flow of information between your computer and any other computer whose number you dial. If your computer came with an internal modem installed, such software almost certainly came installed with it, but you can also choose among many commercial packages. Your best source of advice, other than a knowledgeable friend, is reviews in computer magazines. There's also a specialized class of communications software customized for specific functions, such as making it easier to use a particular information service. For example, chapter 11 is devoted to showing the uses of one such piece of software designed to help search the world's single largest medical database.

TWO TYPES OF INFORMATION RESOURCES: DATA AND PEOPLE

Your computer enhances your ability to reach two kinds of re-sources: documentary materials and other people who can help you.

Documentary materials are found in electronic reference col-lections called *databases*. A database is any searchable collection of information stored in a computer, and an *online* database is one to which you have remote access using a computer equipped with a modem. Examples include the card catalog of a medical li-brary, an index to medical periodicals, or, sometimes, the full text of reference books describing, say, the side effects of drugs. Chapter 10 describes the contents of several major online med-ical databases, beginning with MEDLINE, an immense medical bibliography containing citations and abstracts of articles from medical journals.

You *log on* (connect) to a database by using your communica-tions software to dial its phone number. Once you are connected, an on-screen menu provides basic instructions for using the data-base.

Your actual search for information will be either "menu driven," meaning that you will type brief entries in response to onscreen prompts, or "command driven," meaning that you will type in a series of search commands based on instructions available from the managers of the database. Menu-driven searches are easier be-cause your choices are laid out in front of you; command-driven searches are faster and more flexible. Either way, you'll be able to read on your own screen the contents of the remote database files. In most cases, you can import selected files to your own computer (a process called downloading) and, if you wish, print out your newly acquired information on your own printer.

People who can help are also easy to find online. That's impor-tant because, as wonderful as libraries are, you often have questions that only a live human being can answer. The combination of a personal computer and a telephone enables you to contact far more people than you could conceivably reach otherwise: physicians, the staff of research organizations, reference librarians, and other individuals who may have had to cope at a human level with problems like your own.

How do you locate such people?

Some of them, such as authors of journal articles or directors of organizations, can be identified through careful reading of the materials in online databases. In that sense, scanning a computer screen or printout is no different from reading a printed bibliography.

But a computer also allows you to find helpful people more directly by connecting to online message centers. Imagine, for example, that someone you love has been diagnosed with acoustic neuroma, the inner-ear tumor mentioned in introductory chapters. You want information on the risks and benefits of surgery. Perhaps journal articles haven't completely answered your questions, or perhaps you're not sure that you've found the most important articles. What do you do?

First, find an appropriate message center, such as the CompuServe Cancer Forum. Next, compose your question offline, making it as specific as possible while keeping it succinct. Give it a descriptive title (for example, "Acoustic neuroma — options?") and follow instructions for posting it on the electronic bulletin board. That's all there is to it.

You'll almost certainly get replies. Some correspondents may simply express sympathy and support. Others may mention treatment side effects. You may hear from physicians who'll be willing to explain the meaning of tests, suggest questions to ask your own physician, or mention articles especially worth reading.

A word on terminology may help here. The terms "bulletin board service (BBS)" or simply "board" usually refer to special-purpose message centers reachable by direct dialing; most provide both downloadable reference materials and a board for posting messages. On the Internet, discussed in a separate chapter, these same reference and communication functions are provided through groups variously known as user groups, discussion groups, special interest groups (SIGs), or, often, "lists." Commercial providers of multiple online services may use other names. CompuServe, for example, calls its message boards "Forums," and another vendor calls them "Roundtables." This book uses the terms most common in the context being discussed, but the generic function — to post and reply to messages in a public setting — is the same in all cases.

MAKING DIRECT CONNECTIONS

You can reach many databases and BBSs simply by using your communications software and modem to dial their phone numbers. This is the easiest kind of connection to understand, even if it's not what you may do most often. Many BBSs are oriented toward special problems: AIDS, addiction recovery, particular forms of cancer, vision problems, or physical disabilities. Still others specialize in broad categories of information; for example, pharmacology. Most BBSs contain both message centers and databases, for the same reasons that organizations' offices typically contain specialized libraries.

As a general rule, BBSs do not charge for access or for downloaded information, although some ask for voluntary contributions to defray their owners' expenses. However, only a few BBSs have toll-free numbers, so you can run up a large long-distance phone bill if you stay online for long periods. Note also that some BBSs impose limits on the amount of time per call (or per day) for which you may stay connected.

Unlike bibliographic entries in structured databases like MED-LINE, the files in most BBS libraries are highly variable in their contents. Many of them were uploaded by users like yourself. They may contain the full text of key articles from medical journals, saving you search time and considerable cost. (But remember that these articles will not necessarily be the most recent or targeted to your precise needs.) They may also contain valuable search suggestions, such as lists of *MeSH* subject headings that might not have occurred to you. Other items may include personal opinions, humor, or poetry.

COMMERCIAL ONLINE SERVICES

A commercial online service is likely to prove your single most useful pathway for finding the best treatment, with the possible exception of a direct account with MEDLINE. That's because information in its natural state is scattered, and you'll find it difficult to search every relevant nook and cranny of the online world directly. Commercial online services alleviate this problem by bringing a lot of resources together in one place. As a result, they're sometimes referred to as "information utilities," "information supermarkets," or "information shopping malls." You have to pay for this convenience, of course, just as you pay your telephone company or any other vendor.

Full-service online vendors provide e-mail, message centers, and access to reference materials. The largest of these that provide at least some access to medical materials are America Online, CompuServe, DELPHI, GEnie, and Prodigy. All have their merits. All offer free or nearly free trial periods, so try more than one before making up your mind.

The authors consider CompuServe by far your best choice for serious online medical searches. In many respects, its database access compares to that available on other services as a library compares to a single textbook. Its message centers, which it calls *forums*, are divided into far more special topic areas than those of other vendors. As a result, CompuServe forums attract participants, including physicians and other medical researchers, who tend to be highly focused and able to bring real expertise to answering your inquiries. For these reasons, most of the examples in this book come from CompuServe. Be aware, however, that much of this information exists in databases that you must pay extra to access, so extensive reliance on CompuServe for MEDLINE searches can be expensive.

All consumer-oriented online services are easy to join. For an initial membership fee, the vendor sends communications software tailored to the service, accompanied by instructions for getting started. The membership fee usually entitles you to several free hours of connect time for learning how to use the system. After this trial period, there are as many payment plans as services —

more, actually, since most vendors offer more than one plan. Typically, you may pay any or all of the following:

- a flat monthly rate covering a specified number of hours of connect time;
- per-minute or per-hour charges for connect time in excess of this specified ceiling;
- surcharges, also based on connect time, for access to some of the commercial databases to which the online service offers access;
- fixed fees for additional services, such as downloading (or receiving a faxed copy) of the text of a journal article.

Your monthly fee will entitle you to other services, including electronic mail, or e-mail for short. You can correspond with people who use different vendors than your own, although vendors usually add a surcharge for handling e-mail to and from addresses outside their own systems.

The larger commercial services, like CompuServe and America Online, provide local-call access from almost anywhere in the United States. One caution: although the communications software packages provided by vendors are attractive and easy to use, they may not be designed for maximum efficiency. Like shopkeepers, online vendors make their wares appealing, and they want you to stay online a long time. Nevertheless, a number of third-party software developers have devised ways to reduce your online time. Their customized communications software (often called "front end" packages) make searches faster and more efficient by letting you divide your searches into two separate passes. First, you do a fast scan of a message center's or library's list of contents; then, on your second pass, you retrieve only those items you want to examine. This process makes using online services less like walking aisles of a shopping mall and more like thumbing through a mail-order catalog before placing your order.

Most commercial vendors also offer conference-mode (also called "chat-mode") sessions, in which you and other participants are online at the same time and send typed messages back and forth. The most common purpose of these sessions is social chat, not the exchange of serious information. But an online conference with several people who share your interests can be arranged for less than the cost of a telephone conference call.

FINDING YOUR BEST ACCESS ROUTE TO ONLINE INFORMATION

So what's the *best* way to get from your home computer to databases and bulletin boards?

That depends on your own experience, your finances, and the urgency of your need for information. For most people, however, the following steps should produce the most medical information at the lowest investment in effort, time, and money.

• First, subscribe to a full-service online service that provides e-mail, access to databases, and message centers (forums). Spend at least a few weeks getting to know what the service offers, particularly on its most appropriate forum. Unless your medical problem is very urgent, use services with surcharges sparingly until you know your way around.

• Take full advantage of any free BBS services that pertain to your condition. Remember, however, that you're still paying long-distance telephone charges for information that you *may* be able to download with a local call from a CompuServe forum or other vendor's library at almost no cost.

• For serious searches of clinical literature, register with the National Library of Medicine to get direct access to MEDLINE, whose use is described in later chapters. For anything over minimal use, searching NLM databases directly will be less expensive than going through a commercial vendor.

In short, plan your online expeditions just as you'd plan any travel. Consider your needs, including time pressures, your experience, and your budget. It's nice to know that you can do your learning at 2 A.M., if you need to, well after the kids have gone to bed and long after most libraries are closed.

Finally, just take things a step at a time. If you're starting with no computer experience whatsoever, online searches may sound formidable, just as the recipes in a cookbook can sound formidable to someone who's never cooked. Learning online searching can occasionally, like cooking, be frustrating. Yet once you've made up your mind to become computer literate, you'll learn quickly.

10.

Databases You Should Know About

WHEN VALERIE OSTROTH learned to do online database searching after being diagnosed with chronic fatigue and immune dysfunction syndrome (CFIDS), she could hardly have guessed that these skills would lead to rapid diagnosis and treatment of an acute illness that later struck her father.

The problem began when her parents were away at a conference and her father's nose spontaneously began to discharge a thin, watery fluid. At first they thought the discharge was due to an allergy or the airplane flight. But it persisted, and when he returned home, his primary care physician arranged to have the fluid content checked. Tests of the fluid revealed that it contained glucose, an indicator that it was cerebrospinal fluid, which surrounds the brain and helps protect it from damage.

His physician, unsure of a diagnosis, immediately referred him to a neurologist.

"I went immediately to MEDLINE," Valerie says, "and used 'nose' and 'runny' as search terms. Soon I came up with [a number of articles on] spontaneous cerebrospinal fluid rhinorrhea, which is exactly what my father had."

The neurologist gratefully accepted the printouts of the articles that Valerie had found, noting that the information was more recent than that in his journals. He referred his patient to the University of Virginia hospital, known for innovative approaches to treating this problem. Specialists there, Valerie says, went up through her father's nose and patched the defect at the base of the skull with surgical "super glue." This new procedure probably enabled him to avoid a much more invasive surgical procedure, a craniotomy, which involves removing a portion of the skull and cutting through layers of membranes around the brain.

Valerie notes: "My father's illness was so acute and so potentially life-threatening in so short a time that the information from MEDLINE was priceless . . . From my use of MEDLINE for my father's illness (now cured) and my ongoing CFIDS, I have come to know that I'm not alone and that there *are* places to turn for information."

Valerie's ability to respond with extraordinary speed to a family emergency serves as a reminder that skills in locating information may pay off in unexpected ways. This chapter will introduce you to MEDLINE and a number of other important sources of online data. These databases offer almost immediate access to up-to-date medical information that in many cases cannot be located in any other way. The chapter will also suggest a few general principles applicable to almost all online searches.

AN INTRODUCTION TO MEDLINE

If there's a single database that's indispensable to your search for the best treatment, it's MEDLINE. MEDLINE is the largest single database within a family of online databases collectively known as MEDLARS (MEDical Literature Analysis and Retrieval System). The MEDLARS databases are compiled and maintained by the National Library of Medicine (NLM), which is part of the National Institutes of Health, a federal agency located in Bethesda, Maryland.

MEDLINE is a collection of medical journal citations and abstracts covering virtually every area in the field of biomedicine. It contains well over seven million records from more than 3,800 international biomedical journals, dating from 1966 to the present. More than thirty thousand new citations are added each month. The NLM reports that MEDLINE is searched approximately twenty thousand times per day, mainly by physicians and medical researchers, but often by patients.

Conceptually, MEDLINE resembles the print reference *Index Medicus*. It's a bibliographic database, not a full-text database. But MEDLINE, unlike its print counterpart, does include abstracts for nearly all articles published after 1975, which account for about 70 percent of its citations. MEDLINE is updated weekly (for some types of material), compared to monthly for *Index Medicus*.

For guidance or information, contact NLM at one of the following e-mail addresses:

MEDLARS Service Desk: mms@nlm.nih.gov
Grateful Med: gmhelp@medserv.nlm.nih.gov
Reference Services: ref@nlm.nih.gov

Size and recency apart, you can do things with a computer database that cannot be done with print references, at least not within any reasonable amount of time. Like *Index Medicus*, MEDLINE is indexed by medical subject headings (MeSH) to clarify relationships among different topics and permit someone with a limited medical vocabulary to search MEDLINE with something approaching the effectiveness of a trained librarian. Of course, MeSH doesn't magically empower you with search skills from the instant you sit at a computer keyboard; it does, however, facilitate learning by trial and error. If you think that you may be searching MEDLINE fairly extensively, a direct NLM account is generally less expensive than other options. It's billable to a credit card by contacting the National Library of Medicine, 8600 Rockville Pike, Bethesda, MD 20894. Its toll-free service desk line is (800) 638-8480, and its local number is (301) 496-6193.

An NLM account also provides access to over forty other MEDLARS databases. Searching costs average $18 per hour, but you are billed only for the time you use (on a per-minute basis).

There are no monthly charges or minimum fees. An average search costs only a few dollars, and searches of AIDS-related databases are free. (You will be billed extra if you request a printed copy of the full text of articles, a service for which you must make arrangements with a medical library.)

To use MEDLINE most effectively, purchase a piece of customized communications software called Grateful Med, developed by NLM to make searches of MEDLARS databases easier. If the authors were to select a single software package for you to purchase for your pursuit of the best medical care, it would be this program. With a good medical dictonary, the *Merck Manual*, and Grateful Med, you will have the resources to carry out the vast majority of your searches effectively and at minimum cost. Because of this program's importance, the entire next chapter is devoted to a tutorial on its use.

OTHER WAYS OF REACHING MEDLINE

Instead of a direct-dial connection, you can also reach MEDLINE using local numbers provided by vendors such as Sprint, TYM-NET, or CompuServe. Frequently what sounds like a separate database (for example, a service called Physicians' Online) turns out to be one of many alternative ways of reaching MEDLINE. You can also connect to MEDLINE via the Internet, but you (or the institution through which you connect) will still need an account for searches. Altogether, the NLM has licensed more than eighty commercial vendors and nonprofit institutions in this country and abroad to provide their customers or users with MEDLINE access. If you do not expect to search MEDLINE frequently, you may find it convenient to use one of the vendors. Note, however, that MEDLINE access will usually add a monthly fee to your membership.

With CompuServe, you have three different pathways. The first of these pathways is PaperChase, reachable by typing in the command Go PAPERCHASE. It's a piece of customized communications software resembling Grateful Med in concept, but one that some users prefer. A second CompuServe path to MEDLINE is a bibliographical retrieval service called IQUEST, reachable by typing Go IQUEST. IQUEST provides a uniform format for searching a number of databases, including many in fields unrelated to medicine. The third option for reaching MEDLINE on CompuServe is a bibliographic retrieval service called Knowledge Index, reachable by typing Go KI. Like IQUEST, Knowledge Index contains a great many databases unrelated to medicine. Its medical resources include MEDLINE and several other important databases: Drug Information Fulltext, EMBASE, International Pharmaceutical Abstracts, Mental Health Abstracts, and others.

Searches on either PaperChase or IQUEST can get expensive fast. Their per-hour rates are competitive with NLM MEDLINE searches, but both impose surcharges based on the number of searches you run and the number of abstracts you download. If you want to review a great many abstracts, it's not difficult to run up very substantial bills.

Knowledge Index charges only for connect time (and, of course, special print orders), and its low rates make it a best buy among CompuServe pathways to MEDLINE. But there's one catch. Knowledge Index is available *only* on evenings, weekends, and holidays. If that's not a problem for you, typing "Go KI" on CompuServe won't bankrupt you.

How great are the cost savings using Knowledge Index? One published comparison of costs for hypothetical searches at differing levels of complexity estimated the costs of using IQUEST at from five to ten times the cost of using Knowledge Index, depending on which databases are searched. PaperChase costs tend to approach those of IQUEST.

You should remember also that CompuServe forums contain their own libraries — mini-databases that may include the results of other people's MEDLINE searches. These can be downloaded without paying a surcharge. Scan through those libraries to find files relating to your medical interests collected by other patients or former patients. Be aware, of course, that these files will not necessarily be current and are unlikely to be targeted exactly to your concerns. Think of them as a starting point that can save you time in planning your search strategy.

In summary, CompuServe's prime-time pathways to MED-LINE are expensive, but Knowledge Index provides an economical path to MEDLINE if you can search during evenings and weekends. In general, however, if you search MEDLINE and other MEDLARS databases very often, we recommend a direct account with NLM and the use of Grateful Med. You're billed only for the time you use, so there's little reason not to open an account if you expect to search fairly often.

OTHER NLM DATABASES

MEDLINE is not the only database in the MEDLARS family. There are more than forty of them. The NLM will provide you with a fact sheet describing them and how to reach them, but here are thumbnail sketches of several you should know about. All of them are searchable with Grateful Med (although one of them, PDQ, requires a separate NLM-supplied password). The citations available from a specialized database are (for the most part) also in MEDLINE, but searching a database confined to your interests saves time. For example, searching an AIDS-related database for information on a particular drug will produce only citations on the use of that drug in treating AIDS, not its use in other diseases or conditions.

AIDSLINE (AIDS Information onLINE)

This database contains approximately one hundred thousand bibliographic citations pertaining to acquired immunodeficiency syndrome (AIDS). The records indexed include journal articles (mostly from MEDLINE), government reports, letters, technical reports, monographs, books, audiovisuals, and meeting abstracts. The database is updated weekly and grows at a rate of about nine hundred new entries per month. *Searches on AIDSLINE are free, as are searches on the following two databases.*

AIDSTRIALS and AIDSDRUGS

AIDSTRIALS contains over five hundred records, each covering a single clinical trial of substances being tested for use against AIDS, HIV infection, and AIDS-related opportunistic diseases. The database is updated every two weeks. Each record provides the title and purpose of the trial, the name of the drugs being tested, trial locations, patient eligibility criteria, and the names of contact persons. AIDSDRUGS is a dictionary of chemical and biological agents being evaluated in the trials described in AIDS-TRIALS.

CANCERLIT (Cancer Literature)

CANCERLIT contains about a million bibliographic citations, many of them journal articles from MEDLINE. The file contains government reports, meeting abstracts, monographs, and a few foreign language journals not included in MEDLINE. It also contains articles on the relationship of environmental factors (for example, electromagnetic fields) to cancer.

DIRLINE (DIRectory of Information Resources onLINE)

This is a directory of organizations. The organizations include academic and research institutions, government agencies, information centers, professional societies, and support groups. The records contain the organizations' names, addresses, and phone numbers, plus information on their publications and services.

HSTAR (Health Service/Technology Assessment Research)

HSTAR contains materials both on the development and use of clinical practice guidelines and on technology assessment, taken from MEDLINE and other sources. HSTAR also has meeting abstracts and newspaper articles.

Physician Data Query (PDQ)

PDQ is another cancer-oriented database, maintained by the National Cancer Institute. Rather than bibliographic citations, it contains information about treatments and cancer research in progress. Specifically, it contains detailed descriptions of all major tumor types, the most recent cancer treatments, ongoing investigational and standard protocols, and directories of physicians and organizations involved in state-of-the-art cancer care. There are two versions: one for patients, written in nontechnical language, and one for health professionals. Once armed with a medical dictionary, you will be better off with the reports for professionals. PDQ also has a protocol file containing information on clinical trials of active cancer treatments.

PDQ is not only searchable via Grateful Med but is available at no charge for anyone with Internet access. (It's accessible on the Internet from a "gopher" menu you can reach by typing *gopher helix.nih.gov*.) Note also that PDQ files are regularly transferred to the protocol library of the CompuServe Cancer Forum, from which they can be downloaded without charge.

TOXLINE (TOXicology Information onLINE) and TOXLIT (TOXicology LITerature from Special Sources)

Both of these databases contain bibliographic citations on the effects of drugs and other chemicals. The difference between the two is that the records in TOXLINE are derived from sources that do not charge for information; the entries in TOXLIT come from a commercial database called Chemical Abstracts, whose royalty charges are added to your search costs. In the context of your search for treatment alternatives, only TOXLINE is likely to be of interest, and most of its journal article entries come from MEDLINE.

OTHER ONLINE MEDICAL DATABASES

A great many other medical databases are readily accessible via your home computer. As you become more deeply involved in online searching, particularly by participating in forums on places like CompuServe, America Online, and Prodigy, or perhaps on Internet discussion groups, you will hear about these and other online reference sources. You will also encounter differences of opinion as to how useful a given database is likely to be. Like ordinary libraries, online databases vary with respect both to ease of use and the depth of their holdings.

Like MEDLINE, other databases are typically leased by their developers or owners to various institutions or commercial vendors and may therefore be available at more than one online location. The list of databases that follows is certainly not exhaustive, and some addresses may have changed by the time this is printed. But this list should convey a sense of the kinds of resources available to you.

Black Bag BBS

The Black Bag BBS is a private bulletin board compiled and maintained by Edward Del Grosso, M.D. Reachable by modem at (610) 454-7396, it's an impressive resource, free except for telephone charges. It has a message center resembling those on the major commercial services. Its libraries include files of disease-related information, taken from both published and unpublished sources. For example, the Black Bag includes a section called "AIDS Treatment News" that provides the latest information on AIDS treatment options, updated weekly.

This BBS also has an interactive text-based database that you can search online for a better understanding of diseases, medical procedures, medications, symptoms, and treatments. For example, if you want a nontechnical description of how magnetic resonance imaging (MRI) works, you can find it here. The Black Bag offers the largest available collection of medical software programs in the public domain. You can download any of this software without charge. You can also work through some programs online, such as a cardiopulmonary resuscitation (CPR) tutorial.

One especially useful feature of the Black Bag is its "echo" (reproduction) of messages on more than seventy Internet message centers. This allows you to follow what's available in Internet dis-

cussion groups and contact individuals whose Internet addresses
you know without paying for full Internet access or learning Internet protocols.

The Black Bag provides a guide to roughly four hundred other
medical BBSs. Dr. Del Grosso regularly updates this list, which is
organized by states. It contains names of the BBSs, their phone
numbers, and single-word descriptors of their area of specialization (for example, AIDS, EYES, PSYCH). You can download this
file from the Black Bag itself or from libraries with the MEDSIG
(Medical Special Interest Group) or the CANCER forums on
CompuServe. You can also e-mail a request to an Internet address,
list@blackbag.com. (For an example of one of the BBSs on the Black
Bag list, see the NKCA BBS description below.) For regular users,
other than persons with disabilities, Dr. Del Grosso requests a
modest monetary contribution, either to the Black Bag or to the
Mental Health Association of Collegeville, Pennsylvania.

Comprehensive Core Medical Library (CCML)

CCML offers the most extensive selection of *full-text* (as distinct
from only citations and abstracts) medical journals and reference
works available online. The file contains approximately one hundred of the better-known journals (for example, the *New England
Journal of Medicine*) and key reference works like the *Merck Manual.* You can do a bibliographic search first for citations and abstracts, using online help to locate key words (which are not
identical to MeSH subject headings). CCML is reachable in various ways, including CompuServe (Go CCML).

CompuServe Forum Libraries

CompuServe forum libraries contain extremely valuable reference
materials of many kinds. Among the most important are (1) lists
and addresses of information resources (for example, the Black
Bag list of BBSs); (2) lists of other kinds of resources (for example,
whom to contact at drug companies about the possibility of providing free drugs for people who cannot afford them); (3) free
copies of reference materials for which you'd otherwise have to

pay search charges (for example, searches of MEDLINE by other patients on topics that may interest you); (4) copies of reference materials that you might otherwise have difficulty finding (for example, physician cancer treatment protocols from the NLM-National Cancer Institute's PDQ database); (5) copies of particularly informative message "threads" (sequences of messages on the same topic) that have previously appeared in a forum, and (6) computer programs and routines that can aid you in locating, processing, or displaying online information. (When downloading a *program*, as distinct from a data file, you should check it for computer viruses, using software designed for that purpose.) The exact means of downloading files from CompuServe forums will depend on the communications software you are using.

EMBASE (*Excerpta Medica*)

EMBASE is a giant among databases — on the same order of magnitude as MEDLINE. EMBASE contains much of the same biomedical journal literature as MEDLINE, but it puts more emphasis on drugs and the international pharmaceutical industry. Its records come from over 3,500 journals, over 80 percent of which are indexed cover-to-cover (i.e., the index includes not only articles but reviews, editorials, and letters to editors) and the remainder scanned for drug-related articles. EMBASE, therefore, is one of the few bibliographic databases offering a significant quantity of materials not available on MEDLINE. For example, it includes information on drugs not yet approved for use in the United States. As a result, searches of a single topic on both MEDLINE and EMBASE may produce duplicate citations in a surprisingly small number of cases.

EMBASE is produced by a scientific and technical publishing firm in the Netherlands and is searchable on CompuServe, either through IQUEST or Knowledge Index. For the cost reasons already discussed, Knowledge Index offers the better buy if you can manage non–prime time searches. If you need a search of EMBASE, unless you are prepared to spend time and money learning how to do it efficiently, you may want to consider hiring a professional for this task.

Health Database Plus

This database is reachable in various ways, including a direct pathway on CompuServe (Go HLTDB). Unlike virtually all the other information sources listed in this book, Health Database Plus contains full-text articles on health, medicine, and nutrition from popular magazines, such as *Good Housekeeping, Health*, and *Psychology Today*. It also includes both articles and abstracts from a core set of the best-known technical and professionals journals, such as the *New England Journal of Medicine*. Reading popular medical journalism cannot substitute for reading the primary medical literature, but it may be the easiest way to get an overview of an issue and may often guide you to valuable resources.

Health Database Plus is extremely easy to search by following menu prompts. Other than CompuServe connect time charges, you are billed only for material you actually read, not for citations. But you are charged for any article or abstract you call into view on your screen, whether or not you download it, so you may as well download any text that you ask for.

IQUEST Medical InfoCenter

IQUEST, searchable on CompuServe, has already been mentioned as one path to a number of databases, including MEDLINE and EMBASE. All of its medical databases are collected at one CompuServe address (Go IQMEDICINE). It contains most of the MEDLARS databases (for example, PDQ, AIDS databases, and CANCERLIT). Of particular interest is SciSearch, the online analog of the Science Citation Index mentioned in chapter 6, which provides a way of identifying the institutional affiliations of journal article authors — very useful when you need to contact an expert.

Med Help International

Med Help International is both a database and a search service. A nonprofit corporation, Med Help International was founded and is maintained by Phil Garfinkel and Cynthia Thompson, who became convinced of the need for a service like this after doing their own medical information searches on behalf of family members. You can search the BBS database for information written in nontechnical language; if you don't find what you need, you can request a special report, which will be prepared by a volunteer physician or other health professional. You will be asked to pay $20 per request, but this amount will be reduced or waived altogether if you cannot afford it. The BBS number is (516) 423-0472. E-mail queries may be sent via CompuServe at 73323,3050 or 73174,2405; the Internet address for queries is *philg@world.std.com.* (Med Help International also accepts search questions by phone at (407) 253-9048 or by mail at 6300 N. Wickham Road, Suite 130, Box 188, Melbourne, FL 32940-2029.)

NORD

NORD is the acronym for the National Organization for Rare Disorders, a nonprofit group devoted to dissemination of information on so-called "orphan diseases." NORD defines a rare disease as one affecting fewer than 200,000 Americans, which comes to fewer than one per thousand people. Some of these disorders are considerably rarer than that, and many physicians see them too seldom for easy diagnosis. In fact, the NORD newsletter, *Orphan Disease Update*, asserts that one out of three individuals with a rare disease does not receive a correct diagnosis for up to five years.

The NORD database includes articles on approximately one thousand diseases. Some of these are not rare, but NORD includes them in response to numerous requests for information. The NORD database is available online through CompuServe (Go NORD). You can also send e-mail messages to its research staff at its CompuServe address, 76703,3014 (which becomes *76703.3014@compuserve.com* for people sending messages from other online services). You can also write to NORD, P.O. Box 8923, New Fairfield, CT 06812-8923. If you indicate the disorder that concerns you, the NORD research staff will provide you with a report on the disease. *The first report is free, and subsequent ones are four dollars.*

When you connect to NORD on CompuServe, you'll get a series of menu choices. If you choose to do a search on a particular disease, you'll be given the option of choosing any or all of ten subtopic headings: synonyms, general description, symptoms, causes, affected population, related disorders, therapies (two headings here: "standard" and "investigational"), resources (primarily organizations), and references. The language is nontechnical and unannotated.

NKCA BBS

This is a BBS maintained by the National Kidney Cancer Association (NKCA). It exists mainly for the benefit of individuals with kidney cancer, their families, and professionals involved in kidney cancer research and treatment. Many of its general articles are relevant reading for anyone with cancer of any kind.

A FEW SUGGESTIONS FOR EFFECTIVE SEARCHING

In concept, online searching is no different from searching through print references. Most of your effectiveness will depend on how carefully you select keywords, singly and in combination. It's a good idea to keep notes, not just on what you've found, but on how you got there — including notes on your false starts.

Efficiency is especially important when you're paying for the time you're connected to the database, and still more important when you're paying for the number of items you download. On some databases, floundering around online can be expensive. And, even when you're not being charged for time, it's a courtesy not to tie up a nonprofit service's phone lines for unreasonably long periods. (The founder of one BBS says that callers to his toll-free number cost his organization almost $15 per hour and that its lines handle hundreds of call-in hours per week. This is why many free bulletin boards ration caller connect time.)

The key to efficient online searching is offline planning. In menu-driven databases, in which you select options either by pressing keys or clicking a mouse, you can plunge in and learn as you go, if that's how you learn best. Command-driven databases, in which you must type exact instructions to the host computer, require that you read instructions in advance.

You may have to think creatively in identifying search terms. MEDLINE searches are often more productive if you use *MeSH* subject headings, which can be browsed and selected onscreen and offline using Grateful Med or by consulting print references available in medical libraries. Relatively nontechnical databases, such as those maintained by NORD, CompuServe's Health Database Plus, and various specialized bulletin boards, can be invaluable as a source of leads to recent professional literature.

Many communications software packages permit you to capture an entire online session in a file, and you should take advantage of that feature if you have it. It permits you to review your search when the meter is no longer running and decide what to do differently on the next search.

Most important, you should not be easily discouraged. Even professional searchers routinely make at least two passes through a database — one to get a "feel" for its contents; another to do a careful search based on exact logic and terminology. "Remember that the computer is always there," says Barbara Quint, who edits a magazine for her fellow professional searchers. "Do not try to get every citation you will ever need in the first search. Get some good material. Take it offline and read it. It will probably suggest some alternative search routes to more information. The essence of good search strategy is interactivity. When you own a well, you don't need to drink by the bucketful. One glass at a time."

Valerie Ostroth agrees.

"People who are afraid to use the computer," she says, "should start simply. People have to find their own little corner and experiment."

11.

A MEDLINE Search Using "Grateful Med"

MICHAEL CODY WAS used to it. People had asked him for help like this before. Now, his friend Bill was telling him that his wife, who had been diagnosed with non-Hodgkin's lymphoma (a cancer of the lymphatic system) was so sick from chemotherapy that she was thinking of dropping out of treatment. She was taking an anti-nausea drug, but it didn't seem to be working. Bill was wondering if Michael could find out if there were other anti-nausea drugs available that he might ask her doctor about at their next appointment.

That night, Michael sat before his computer, connected to MEDLINE through his Grateful Med communications program, and typed in some key words, such as "nausea," "chemically induced," and "prevention and control." Soon he came up with a number of article citations and abstracts (summaries) — many of them about a new, highly effective class of antiemetic (anti-nausea) drugs.

At their next appointment, Bill and his wife took the article abstracts about the new class of drugs to the doctor. The doctor said he was aware of the new drugs and had been considering trying them in the near future, but would be willing to begin right then.

Soon, the new regimen was successfully controlling the vomiting. Bill's wife was now able to handle her chemotherapy sessions, and no longer thought of quitting.

As another searcher has said, the thirty-dollar price of Grateful Med is "a pauper's sum for a princely product."

Knowing how to find medical journal citations and abstracts in the huge bibliographic database MEDLINE is central to your search for the best treatment. Because it's so important, this chapter walks you through the process of searching MEDLINE using the communications software package called Grateful Med. Although there are many ways to reach MEDLINE and many packages for searching it, Grateful Med is, for most personal computer users, the most easily accessible and least expensive choice.

Grateful Med is available from National Technical Information Service (NTIS), 5285 Port Royal Road, Springfield, VA 22161. If you pay by credit card, you can order by phone at (800) 423-9255 without shipping and handling charges. The order number for the IBM-DOS version is PB92-105444/GBB; for the Macintosh version, it's PB93-502433. (A Windows version is promised shortly and may be available by the time you read this.) If you're undecided, NLM will provide a free demonstration disk of Grateful Med. The NLM also offers an array of print, audiovisual, and computer-based reference tools, including aids to searching MEDLINE and other databases, described in a free publications catalog available from NLM.

AN OVERVIEW OF THE SEARCH PROCESS

This chapter focuses on searches of MEDLINE, but most of it also applies to searching other NLM databases.

First, here's a bird's-eye view of the whole process, based on the DOS version.

The first time you run Grateful Med (by typing the command SEARCH), the first screen you see on your monitor identifies the product, and then shifts you into a SETUP program. You next enter local phone numbers, an account number, and a password, all supplied by NLM. The instructions are clear.

On subsequent runs, you'll quickly reach a screen headed "Select the ACTION you want to take." From here on we'll call this the Action screen. (This and other screens mentioned in this overview will be displayed later in the chapter to illustrate an actual search.) The Action screen offers several choices, any of which may be selected by moving the screen cursor to the appropriate line and pressing ENTER.

After you choose MEDLINE, a screen headed INPUT YOUR SEARCH appears. If you're looking for a particular author or title, type those entries into the labeled blanks, or else leave those lines blank and do a subject search. That's when Grateful Med begins to demonstrate that computer-assisted searching isn't just ten times *faster* than using print references like *Index Medicus*; it's also *smarter*, enabling you to improve your chances of finding what you need.

It's better not to type in your own first guess at a subject heading. Instead, get into the habit of tapping the F10 key on your keyboard. This calls up MEDLINE's list of keywords, known as MeSH (for Medical Subject Headings) — the same system whose print version is described in chapter 5.

MeSH will help you choose search terms with precision — a major asset. Remember, a computer is like a fussy clerk who may give you no information at all (or more information than you can handle, which is just as bad) if you don't ask for what you want in the way it's been instructed to serve you.

After you press F10, a screen will appear describing MeSH and asking for the first few letters of where you want to look in its list of keywords. For example, if you're interested in breast cancer, type BREAST. You'll immediately be shown a range of choices, from BREAST, CYST to BREAST, XERORADIOGRAPHY. Grateful Med will also suggest that you check entries under MAMMA- and MAST-. In the unlikely event that you can't find an appropriate MeSH term, you can always go back to the INPUT YOUR SEARCH menu and type in your own best guess.

After making your selections, check how your subject entries appear on your screen. Two subject entries on a single line are the equivalent of a logical OR, meaning that you'll get everything on either subject. For example, if you search MASTECTOMY *OR* POSTOPERATIVE COMPLICATIONS, you'll get not only all mastectomy entries but also every entry on the postoperative complications of any surgery of any kind, head to toe. Entering subject entries on separate lines (up to four are available), such as MASTECTOMY *AND* POSTOPERATIVE COMPLICATIONS, narrows the search to citations that fit both headings.

You can narrow a search further — for example, to only English-language articles or to review articles. You can broaden a search by going back further in time than Grateful Med's default choice of articles published within the past three years. (A *default* choice is a selection that the program assumes when you don't specify otherwise.) Near the bottom of the screen, a prompt asks if you want to see abstracts. On your first pass, say "no"; you'll still get full citations and lists of keywords under which each citation is indexed.

So far, all this has been done offline, meaning before your computer makes connection with the NLM host computer where MEDLINE is stored. You can still go back and make changes in your search criteria. But when Grateful Med prompts OK TO GO ON TO SEARCH? and you type "Y," for "yes," you'll hear buzzing and clicking as your modem dials MEDLINE. If all goes normally, this will be followed by a screen display of those coded greetings that computers exchange whenever they meet. Soon your search results will scroll by on screen, faster than you can read them. When the complete results are entered into your computer, Grateful Med will hang up your phone and shut down your modem.

Your search results are saved automatically to your computer's hard disk. You can review them and, if you wish, save them to a permanent file. (Otherwise, they'll be erased the next time you go online.) You can modify your search criteria for other passes at MEDLINE. If you know you want a particular article, you can ask for its abstract by a unique item number that will appear with its citation.

If your search was an average one, its cost was about $1.25 —

billable to a credit card. The exact amount depends mainly on time online, which in turn depends on how many hits (records matching your search criteria) your search produced and whether you asked for abstracts as well as citations.

A SAMPLE SEARCH IN MORE DETAIL

Now let's run through an actual sample search in more detail.

Consider the worst possible case with respect to knowing where to start a search. You don't know the name of your medical problem — only your symptoms. Although you should never try to diagnose yourself, a MEDLINE search could help you identify possibilities that your physician may not have considered.

Recall that Gayle Allison suffered for *ten years* before her inner ear tumor, known as an acoustic neuroma, was correctly diagnosed. Her symptoms included ringing in the ears, later followed by one-sided hearing loss and dizziness. Suppose that you've had similar symptoms and no idea what might be causing them. Here's how a possible search on your symptoms might progress.

Type the command SEARCH, pressing the ENTER key on your keyboard, and proceed until you reach the screen headed "Select the ACTION you want to take." (See Figure 11-1. All screen simulations are from the DOS version of Grateful Med.)

Select the Action screen's first choice, "MEDLINE — Search biomedical journals." That brings up the screen headed INPUT YOUR SEARCH. (Figure 11-2. Grateful Med's online help instructions refer to this as the "Form" screen, so that's what it'll be called here.) Note that pressing F3 will give you a chance to search further back in time than Grateful Med's default of three years.

By striking TAB or ENTER, move the cursor to the line that provides space for typing in AUTHOR NAME. Since you don't even have a name for the disorder that's troubling you, you certainly don't have an author or title in mind. Leave this line and the next one, TITLE WORDS, blank.

When you reach the line marked SUBJECT WORDS, your first impulse may be to type in something like "ringing in the ears." There's a better, more systematic way. Press the F10 key. A screen, sufficiently clear so as not to require showing it here, describes MeSH and asks you to enter (near its upper right corner) the first several letters, up to ten, of a word you think may be a good search term.

Try "ringing."

Unfortunately, this particular guess leads to keywords such as "Ring Chromosomes," "Ring Constrictions, Intrauterine," "Ringworm," and even "Monkey, Ring-Tail." None of these looks helpful. That's because "ringing in the ears" doesn't happen to be a label on the electronic file drawer where information on that particular symptom is stored.

Searching for New Keywords

For a fresh start, make a list of ordinary English words that might pertain to your condition — e.g., "ear," "deafness," "buzzing," and "hearing." "Hearing" seems both descriptive and general, so start with it. Use the ESCAPE key to get back to the INPUT YOUR SEARCH screen. Next, press F10 and enter the word "hearing," or "Hearing." Grateful Med is not case-sensitive.

The alphabetic MeSH keyword search screen on which "Hearing" entries appear looks like Figure 11-3. A long list of "Hearing" entries appears just under "Healthy Worker Effect." You could enter "Hearing" as a search term, but that would obviously be casting your net far too widely. Several entries, such as "Hearing Loss, Partial," are followed by a "+" symbol. This symbol indicates that the word represents a relatively broad category that contains subcategories.

Several of these keywords look promising, but to get the broadest possible perspective before pursuing any one lead intensively, it's a good idea to examine entries under the major synonyms for "Hearing." These are "Audio-" and "Acoustic." Instructions at the bottom of the screen explain that typing "E" (for "Elsewhere") will give you the opportunity to enter new search terms. Note also that within MeSH the ENTER key is used as a toggle switch to select or deselect a keyword.

Typing "E" and entering the new search term "Audio-" brings up subheadings like "Audiology," "Audiometry," and "Audio-

Select the »ACTION« you want to take

MEDLINE	– Search biomedical journals.
OTHER	– Search other databases.
DIRECT	– Search directly (MEDLARS, TOXNET, PDQ, HES).
AGAIN	– Rerun last search.
REVIEW	– Redisplay results of previous search.
USE	– Retrieve user search file.
EXPLAIN	– See GRATEFUL MED system description.
SETUP	– Enter new telephone numbers or parameters.
LOANSOME	– Order documents.
QUIT	– Exit to DOS.

USE THE ARROW KEYS TO HIGHLIGHT YOUR CHOICE AND PRESS ENTER.
OR ENTER THE FIRST LETTER OF THE HIGHLIGHTED TERM

Figure 11-1. Grateful Med's "Action" screen, with the option of searching MEDLINE highlighted.

```
            INPUT YOUR SEARCH          (1992-1995)  MEDLINE

FILL IN ONLY THE LINES YOU NEED FOR YOUR SEARCH.
PRESS  HOME  FOR HELP;  ESC  TO RESTART;  F1  TO INCLUDE OLDER MATERIAL.

AUTHOR NAME

TITLE WORDS

SUBJECT WORDS

2ND SUBJECT

3RD SUBJECT

4TH SUBJECT

ENGLISH ONLY

  PUBL TYPE

JOURNAL ABBREV
```

Figure 11-2. Grateful Med's "Form" screen, used to enter search parameters prior to launching a MEDLINE search.

```
┌─────────────────────────────────────────────────────────────────┐
│                    Alphabetic MeSH Terms                          │
├───────────────────────────────────────────────────────────────────┤
│ Hearing  + [consider also terms at ACOUSTIC and AUDIO-]           │
│ Hearing  Aids +                                                    │
│ Hearing  Disorders +                                               │
│ Hearing  Loss, Bilateral                                           │
│ Hearing  Loss, Central                                             │
│ Hearing  Loss, Conductive                                          │
│ Hearing  Loss, Extreme (xr) [=Deafness +]                         │
│ Hearing  Loss, Functional                                          │
│ Hearing  Loss, High-Frequency                                      │
│ Hearing  Loss, Noise-Induced                                       │
│ Hearing  Loss, Nonorganic (xr) [=Hearing Loss, Functional]        │
│ Hearing  Loss, Partial +                                           │
│ Hearing  Loss, Sensorineural +                                     │
│ Hearing  Protective Devices (xr) [=Ear Protective Devices]        │
│ Hearing  Tests +                                                   │
│ Rehabilitation of  Hearing   Impaired + [automatic +; always includes more ↩] │
│ Heart + [general: consider specific parts or+ for all             │
│ Heart + cont: consider also terms at CARDI- and MYOCARDI-]        │
│                                                                    │
│  ┌────────────────────────────────────┐   ┌──────────────────────┐ │
│  │ ENTER  Select/Deselect    E Go elsewhere │ │↓↑ PgDn/Up Move Cursor│ │
│  │  +  Plus specific terms   F5 See specific terms │ │← → View rest of term │ │
│  │  *  Major concept only                   │ │HOME   Help           │ │
│  └────────────────────────────────────┘   └──────────────────────┘ │
│         ▲            ESC - Return to Form Screen                   │
└───────────────────────────────────────────────────────────────────┘
```

Figure 11-3. Grateful Med's screen showing alphabetic MeSH search terms under the general category "Hearing." Terms followed by a "+" symbol contain subcategories, viewable by pressing the F5 key.

visual," suggesting that the word usually refers to "sound" rather than "hearing." Make a mental note of this and press on. "Acoustic" is intriguing but equally unhelpful at this point. Its subheadings under "Acoustic Nerve +" include "Acoustic Nerve Diseases +" and references to specific disorders, including "Acoustic Neuroma." But under the assumptions we've made so far, that term doesn't mean anything special to you at this point. Type "E" and enter "hearing."

Back under "Hearing +," "Hearing Disorders +" and "Hearing Loss, Partial +" seem the most promising lines to pursue. It's easy to check both, but "Hearing Loss, Partial +" matches your symptoms of one-sided hearing loss. When you press F5 next (per the instructions at the bottom of the screen), you get a screen labeled "More Specific MeSH Terms — Level 1" (Figure 11-4).

Note that the screen shown as Figure 11-4 lists five possible search terms referring to different kinds of partial hearing loss: "Bilateral," "Conductive," "Functional," "High-Frequency," and "Sensorineural." Even after checking their meanings in your medical dictionary, you may have no sure way of knowing which might apply to your condition, so keep *all* of "Hearing Loss, Partial +" as a search category. Select it by pressing ENTER and then press ESCAPE until you're returned to the "Form" screen, where the words "Hearing Loss, Partial +" now appear in the first SUBJECT WORDS line. This term becomes your first search parameter.

Because MeSH is cross-indexed, you might have arrived at this same point by any of several other routes. For example, instead of "Hearing" you might have entered "Deafness," or, for that matter, "Ear." Working your way through subentries under either "Deafness" and "Ear, Diseases of" would have led you eventually to "Hearing Loss, Partial +."

In hopes of finding a second keyword to narrow your search, check under the other promising MeSH category, "Hearing Disorders +." Its subcategories prove to be "Deafness +" (probably too broad), "Hearing Loss, Partial +" (which you've already chosen), "Recruitment," and "Tinnitus." Let's assume that the latter two terms are unfamiliar. A medical dictionary says that "recruitment" refers to a sensory organ's overreacting to a stimulus — in

```
                    More Specific MeSH Terms - Level 1

▶ Hearing Loss, Partial +
      Hearing Loss, Bilateral
      Hearing Loss, Conductive
      Hearing Loss, Functional
      Hearing Loss, High-Frequency
      Hearing Loss, Sensorineural +


 ENTER  Select/Deselect      F6  Up one level         ↑↓ PgDn/Up  Move Cursor
   +  Plus specific terms     F5  See specific terms   ←→  View rest of term
   *  Major concept only                               HOME Help
              ESC - Return to Alphabetic MeSH
```

Figure 11-4. Subcategories of the **MeSH** term "Hearing Loss, Partial +." This list appears after you move a cursor to "Hearing Loss, Partial +" on the alphabetic **MeSH** terms screen (Figure 11-3) and press the key.

the case of the ear, producing an impression of "loudness." Interesting, but it doesn't fit your symptoms. Now try "Tinnitus." It means "noise inside the ears."

"Tinnitus," therefore, is the medical name for one of your symptoms and appears an excellent choice for your second search term. Be careful, however, not to add it to the first SUBJECT WORDS line, along with "Hearing Loss, Partial +." Recall that Grateful Med considers two entries on a single line to mean a logical "OR." You'd get every citation on both topics. Instead, move the cursor down to the 2ND SUBJECT line and press F10 to call up MeSH again. Type in something like TINN to bring up "Tinnitus" on the alphabetic list of keywords. Mark it on the screen by pressing ENTER, then press ESCAPE, so that MeSH can enter it on the 2ND SUBJECT line of the SEARCH screen.

Why go back into MeSH when you already know that "Tinnitus" is the word you want? Why not just type it in yourself? You could do that, but relying on MeSH is preferable. First, you might make an error typing in "Tinnitus." Grateful Med won't. Second, there may be adjacent entries on the MeSH keyword list you'll want to see. Third, and perhaps most important, you can type in only single-word terms without risking distortions in your search logic. Although "Tinnitus," a single word, doesn't pose this problem, other terms would. For example, trying to type in the two-word term "variant angina" results in a dual entry, "variant OR angina," which would produce all records under "angina" and a no doubt immense number under "variant." MeSH, by contrast, leads to a precise MEDLINE search term, "Angina pectoris, variant." (The only time you might use two MeSH entries on one line is when you want all citations for two fairly precise and related terms, such as "Hearing Loss, Noise-Induced" and "Hearing, Protective Devices.")

Since "Hearing Loss, Partial +" and "Tinnitus" seem reasonable keywords for an exploratory search, skip over the third and fourth SUBJECT lines by pressing ENTER. Next, since understanding unfamiliar medical literature will be a sufficient challenge in English, accept the ENGLISH ONLY restriction by pressing any character key. If you wanted to see articles in other languages, you'd TAB past this entry.

Finally, the menu offers a wide range of choices pertaining to PUBLICATION TYPE. On a first pass, either accept everything or, if the subject you're searching is very broad, consider limiting it to review articles. For this session, press ENTER twice to allow all publication types and journals. As suggested earlier, answer "No" to the prompt inquiring whether you want abstracts. You don't know yet how many articles Grateful Med is going to locate under the headings you've picked. Your first search may yield hundreds of hits, and recovering that many abstracts wastes time. (If you do order abstracts and start getting more than you want to pay for, don't panic. After displaying fifty records, Grateful Med will stop and ask if you wish to continue or quit. So any actual damage to your pocketbook will be limited.)

Now Grateful Med asks if you're ready to do the search. Assume that you decide, on a last-minute hunch, that you wish to search over the most recent seven-year period, instead of Grateful Med's default of three years. Press "N," which returns your cursor to the top of the page, then press F3, which calls up a screen that asks you to add years to the default option. Type in "4" and press ENTER to select the additional years, and then press END to return to the Form screen. Finally, move the cursor down again to the line that asks if you're ready to search. Your Form screen now looks like Figure 11-5 (except that the dates may differ).

This time, press "Y" and ENTER. Within a few seconds, you're connected to MEDLINE. An onscreen greeting will warn you not to worry about how fast information scrolls past. Then, almost before you realize it, your first search is completed. You're told that your search resulted in the selection of 18 records.

A screen message tells you how long you were connected to MEDLINE and what the search cost. (Doing the search described above required 24 seconds online and cost $.87. If you were to repeat the identical process, you might get slightly different results if new items have been added to MEDLINE.)

Grateful Med also permits examining search results in more detail. Use the ESCAPE key to return to the Action screen and choose the option "USE — Retrieve user search file." (Avoid con-

FILL IN ONLY THE LINES YOU NEED FOR YOUR SEARCH.
PRESS **HOME** FOR HELP; **ESC** TO RESTART; **F3** TO INCLUDE OLDER MATERIAL.

AUTHOR NAME

TITLE WORDS   ↓ ENTER TITLE WORDS.

SUBJECT WORDS   ↓ ENTER WORDS, F10 FOR MESH, OR F7 FOR RELEVANT TERMS.
                         explode Hearing Loss, Partial
         and   ↓ ENTER ALTERNATIVE WORDS FOR NEXT CONCEPT, IF ANY.
2ND SUBJECT   Tinnitus (th)
         and   ↓ ENTER ALTERNATIVE WORDS FOR NEXT CONCEPT, IF ANY.
3RD SUBJECT

4TH SUBJECT

ENGLISH ONLY   ↓ ENTER ANY CHARACTER TO SEARCH ONLY ENGLISH LANGUAGE.
                         English Only.
         and   ↓ PRESS F10 FOR LIST OR ANY CHARACTER FOR REVIEWS ONLY.
PUBL TYPE

JOURNAL ABBREV   ↓ ENTER JOURNAL ABBREVIATION. USE F10 KEY FOR LIST.

                         DO YOU WANT TO RETRIEVE THE ABSTRACTS ? (y/N/o) N
                         OK TO GO ON TO SEARCH ? (Y/n/v/s/**)

Figure 11-5. The "Form" screen as it appears at the starting point of a MEDLINE search based on the subject terms "Hearing Loss, Partial +" and "Tinnitus" and covering the years 1992 –1995. (The word "explode" on the SUBJECT WORDS line means "include all subheadings," indicated elsewhere by a "+.") Only English-language articles will be cited — without abstracts. There are no limits on type of publication.

fusing this USE command with REVIEW, which allows you to review the actual citations saved from any previous search.) The USE option calls up your last Form screen again, this time with the number of hits displayed next to each entry. The search just completed found 727 records under "Hearing Loss, Partial +" and 406 records under "Tinnitus." However, only 25 records contained *both* keywords, and of these only 18 (those published in English) were accepted.

Eighteen abstracts is a manageable number to review, so repeat the search, but this time select "Y" for downloading abstracts. It is helpful to have a look at all of them before changing anything in the search design. Downloading all 18 abstracts (each a page or so in length) takes longer than the first search — 3 minutes, 48 seconds. As a result, costs are a little higher — but still only $3.26.

Follow the onscreen prompts to review and save your search results. You should, of course, save the search you've just done under a file name that will help you remember what's in it. Otherwise, Grateful Med erases the most recent search result when it makes a new one.

To save your search on a citation-by-citation basis, select "F" ("write to File"). Select "CTRL-F" for the citation you see on your screen plus all subsequent ones. (If you are looking at citation number 12, for example, CTRL-F will save 12 and all numbers after that, but *not* numbers 1–11.) You'll be prompted to enter a file name and can, if you wish, specify a drive or directory on your computer — for example, A: ACOUST01. Grateful Med provides a file extension automatically. After entering the file name, select the format. It's generally best to accept the default MEDLARS (TAGGED), which will show a REV extension after your file, as in A:ACOUST01.REV. This will permit you to review references later within Grateful Med by using the REVIEW option on the Action screen. Selecting the alternative format (shown onscreen as GRATEFUL MED) will require you to use a word-processing package to look at or print the file.

To print a reference directly from the screen, type "P," followed at the prompt by "Y." Grateful Med may wait for possible further selections or a "CTRL-P." "CTRL-P" functions like "CTRL-F";

that is, it results in printing out the reference on your screen and all subsequent ones.

FOLLOWING UP ON YOUR INITIAL SEARCHES

For those needing to narrow or expand a search, Grateful Med offers suggestions for change — typically by date, by added subject term, or by type of journal. It's a good idea to change only one factor per search and to keep a written record of what you've done. Without good notes, you're likely to find yourself repeating previous passes.

What you do at this point will depend on your own situation — specifically, the information resources at your disposal.

As you review your search so far, you see that the abstracts contain technical words. Since you are unlikely to be familiar with all of them, you'll need a medical dictionary. But a glance at how articles are cross-referenced shows that tinnitus can be a symptom of any of several problems: temporomandibular joint syndrome (commonly known as TMJ), Meniere's disease (a disease of the inner ear), an acoustic neuroma, and others.

Neither Grateful Med nor any other computer program can tell you whether your tinnitus and your partial hearing loss are caused by TMJ, an acoustic neuroma, or something else. Computer programs do exist for use by doctors to aid in diagnosis, but even if you should happen to have access to such a program, you should not risk self-diagnosis or self-treatment of a potentially serious condition.

Bear in mind, however, that you've just explored Grateful Med under the least-promising conditions — when you didn't have a clue what your illness might be. As you read further, you'll master a new vocabulary and be able to ask sharper and sharper questions.

Assume now, for example, that a physician has correctly diagnosed you as having an acoustic neuroma but has mentioned only conventional surgery as a treatment option. You can use Grateful Med to search MEDLINE to see if other options are available.

By a process similar to the one already described, you might use

MeSH keyword listings within Grateful Med and go from "Surgery +" to "Surgical Techniques +." Combining "Surgical Techniques +" with "Acoustic Neuroma" leads to a number of entries, including second-level subheadings that include "Stereotactic Surgery," "Radiosurgery," and "Gamma Knife." That discovery in itself tells you that these are alternatives to conventional surgery; reading the abstracts and later the articles will tell you that they are alternatives worth your serious attention. For example, you might want to consider the following (condensed) citation:

UI — 92334891 [UI stands for "unique identifier," an order number.]

AU — Lunsford LD

TI — Stereotactic radiosurgery in the treatment of patients with acoustic tumors.

RF — REVIEW ARTICLE: 54 REFS.

AD — Department of Neurological Surgery, University of Pittsburgh School of Medicine, Pennsylvania. [AD stands for "Author data."]

MH — *Microsurgery [MH stands for Medical Heading. The asterisk means this is a primary keyword; the full list of keywords on this article is about twenty words long. Only two others are shown here.]

MH — Radiosurgery/ADVERSE EFFECTS/CONTRA-INDICATIONS/*METHODS

MH — Treatment Outcome

PT — REVIEW [PT stands for Publication Type.]

LA[nguage] — Eng

SO[urce] — Otolaryngol Clin North Am 1992 Apr;25 (2):471–91

The title of this article suggests that the procedure "stereotactic radiosurgery" may offer a promising alternative to conventional surgery. As a result, this is a reference for which you'll almost certainly want to see at least the abstract and probably the full text. A procedure for obtaining a copy of the full text is discussed later in this chapter.

DIRECT MEDLINE SEARCHING

If you prefer to search MEDLINE without using Grateful Med's menu prompts, you can select the DIRECT option on the initial Action screen. If you choose this route, you should order *The Basics of Searching MEDLINE*, for $25.50. Remember that it's especially important to plan any direct search strategy offline, while the meter isn't running.

Before you go online, also consider consulting *Permuted Medical Subject Headings*, which takes each significant word from every MeSH subject heading and lists it alphabetically, then lists all the headings in which that word appears. Seeing these possible connections across subject lines may suggest new ideas for searches.

When you choose the DIRECT option, a menu appears that offers several options, including a search of PDQ (Physician's Data Query), which lists cancer treatments and investigational protocols. Assuming that you choose MEDLINE/MEDLARS, Grateful Med will dial up MEDLINE just as it did before, but this time no text will whiz by onscreen. You'll have to type in commands. Moreover, you won't have such quick and easy access to MeSH.

Why might you want to go this route rather than use Grateful Med's menus? The main advantage of a command search is that you can try different combinations of keywords online, see how many hits you get, and make immediate decisions about narrowing or expanding your search. When you already know the keywords you want, direct searches take less of your time, even if you spend a few extra seconds online typing in instructions. Direct searches also enable you to sharpen your search focus with a logical AND NOT function, as in MASTECTOMY *AND* POSTOPERATIVE COMPLICATIONS, *AND NOT* RECONSTRUCTIVE SURGERY. The AND NOT command is omitted from the automated Grateful Med search menu.

Whatever search strategy you select, it's unlikely that you'll satisfy all your MEDLINE information needs in one session at a computer terminal. Your search for the most relevant journal articles is far more likely to be a series of steps.

GETTING COPIES OF ARTICLES USING "LOANSOME DOC"

If you're fortunate enough to live near a good medical library, you may be able to find some of the journals you want on the shelves, or your librarian may be able to get articles for you under an interlibrary loan arrangement.

Even if you live far from a medical library, however, Grateful Med enables you order photocopies of articles, using a feature called "Loansome Doc." The pun may be strained, but the service is excellent. With only a few, one-time preliminary steps, you'll be able to set up the equivalent of a personalized interlibrary loan system accessible from your home computer.

To make use of the interlibrary services of the NLM, you will need an agreement with an "ordering library" that provides Loansome Doc support. Ordering libraries use the NLM's automated interlibrary loan request and referral system, called DOCLINE. To find one near you, call (800) 338-RMLS (7657) and press '1' to be automatically connected to your regional library.

Your regional library may give you more than one library to choose from. Unless you want to pick up articles in person — rather than have them sent by mail or fax — the ordering library you choose can be anywhere in your region. The kind of billing service arrangement you're offered may dictate your choice. Each library has its own set of rules for billing. In some cases, it will simply send an ordinary invoice once a month or as necessary. In others, a credit card number is required, and in some cases, the library will ask you to set up a deposit fund, against which charges will be made. All libraries will send you a contract to sign, stating the method by which you will pay for documents. Prices range from about eight to twenty-five dollars per article sent by mail, and roughly twice as much for fax transmittals.

Once your regional library provides you with the names and phone numbers of possible "ordering libraries" and you've decided which to call, contact a reference library for the information about their service. After you have returned the signed contract to your ordering library, the librarian there will provide you with the library's identifying number, which you'll need to enter when you first set up Loansome Doc. To set up, select "Loansome Doc Configuration Screen" and follow the prompts to enter name, address, library identification number, and so forth.

You select the articles you want through Loansome Doc while reviewing Grateful Med search results by pressing "O" ("Select to Order"). A message at the top of the screen will show that you've tagged that document to order. After completing the review, the "Select Next Step" screen will display a menu of choices. Select "Loansome Doc Actions" and then "Order" ("Send Order to Your Library.") The whirring sounds of your modem connecting will be followed by your "Loansome Doc" Action screen displaying the message "Your Orders Were Sent Successfully." You'll have your articles in the mail in anywhere from a few days to — in some cases — about three weeks. If you've selected the option of receiving them by fax, you'll of course save time. Whenever you'd like to see the status of your Loansome Doc order, select "Review Last Loan Status Report" from the Loansome Doc screen.

Many public libraries offer interlibrary loan retrieval of medical journal articles. There is usually a photocopying fee, and it generally takes a few weeks to receive the articles. If you have Grateful Med software, however, the Loansome Doc option is often a better choice. Chapter 6 describes still other document delivery options.

If you're particularly eager to lay your hands on the full text of an article and nothing seems fast enough, contact a reference librarian at your ordering or regional library. Give the citation of the article and ask the librarian if that journal is in the library's collection, or if not, whose collection might have it. In cases of emergency, the librarian may be willing to help you make some special arrangement to receive a photocopy.

12.

Human Contacts
by Computer

"MY MOM IS the one who helped us get this computer," Valerie Brown, who lives in Maumee, Ohio, says. "When we got home and told her the good news, she actually kissed the thing!"

Although the good news was to prove temporary, the Brown family needed it. Early in 1994, Val's husband, Mike, had been diagnosed with colon cancer — a cancer whose spread would, somewhat over a year later, prove fatal. Yet it was amazing to Val then, and remains a comfort to her, that a computer bought merely for entertainment had enabled her to locate a group of oncologists at Ohio State University Medical School who considered Mike a potential survivor and who treated him accordingly.

When tests showed that Mike's cancer had spread beyond his colon to other parts of his body, the Browns understood that Mike's condition was serious. Valerie especially hated the feeling of helplessness fostered by Mike's oncologist's less-than-aggressive search for treatment options.

During the summer of 1994, however, the Browns acquired a computer. Valerie's mother thought that playing games on it would help occupy Mike's mind.

"The main reason I wanted one," Val says, "was that I'd heard about the Internet and all of this wonderful, vast amount of information you can find. I wanted to dig in and see if I could do any research for him."

She'd seldom used a computer and had never used one to search for information over telephone lines.

"I joined CompuServe," she says, "because in the brochure it said something specifically about a Cancer Forum. And I'll tell you, it took me a good week before I got the courage even to enter the Forum."

Almost immediately, however, she found a sympathetic mentor, a woman who coached her in locating information. Val was astonished to discover that there were physicians on the Cancer Forum who, while declining to diagnose or prescribe, would answer technical questions. Her new friend also mentioned someone thoroughly familiar with the cancer treatment facilities at Ohio State University Medical School. Val and Mike made inquiries and decided to arrange for a consultation. After a battery of tests, a full discussion of options, and a decision on a new course of chemotherapy, the Browns returned home encouraged.

"The people there were just incredible," Val says. "You know, my husband looked fantastic and felt pretty good throughout all of this. They made an issue of that down there. Their attitude is that there's always something else to try. Mike said, 'I feel like a patient now, and not a guinea pig.'"

Mike died of cancer in the spring of 1995, so the Browns' search for treatment options can't be counted a success story of the kind described in earlier chapters of this book. Yet Val remains impressed by the speed with which she located both information and new friends online. She's also glad to have been able to help Mike "fight like hell" during the last months of his life, rather than succumb to despair.

WHAT ONLINE MESSAGE CENTERS CAN DO FOR YOU

That experience illustrates one of the things that your personal computer, connected to a modem, can help you do. Previous chapters have emphasized access to databases, that is, to library-like collections of information. But you also need access to people — both experts who can help you interpret medical information and individuals who have firsthand knowledge of what you're experiencing.

This chapter introduces you to a sample of online message boards, suggests how you can get the most benefit from them, and mentions a few potential problems and how to avoid them. Online message centers aren't *organizations*. You don't join anything, and you're unlikely to get on a permanent mailing list by contacting them. There are no regular meetings to attend. Although many participants are "regulars," people come and go as they please. In fact, it's not easy to decide whether these message boards are best described as "centers," "groups," or "mini-networks." In any case, they provide a convenient and often highly effective way for you to expand and focus your search for the best treatment.

THE COMPUSERVE CANCER FORUM

The CompuServe Cancer Forum provides a sophisticated example of an online message board. It began in 1988, after the mother of its founder, John Ross, complained that the phones at a local cancer information hotline were always busy when she called for advice on *her* mother's illness. Ross recalls: "I said it was a shame the hotline wasn't on CompuServe, as the lines there are seldom busy. The proverbial light bulb lit up. . . ."

Today, the Cancer Forum has about 9,500 members worldwide. It offers a library (database), a message area or bulletin board, and a "conference room" in which up to 150 people can type notes back and forth more or less simultaneously (the online equivalent of a conference call). The library stores files about various kinds of cancers, computer programs that aid searching other databases, and archives consisting of past message threads. (In the language of online message centers, a "thread" is a message and the replies to it, including any additional questions or comments the original sender may later add.) You can scan text files online if you wish, or you can download them for printing.

There's a lot of free material here imported from other databases. For example, the library includes all of the current PDQ (Physician's Data Query) files from the National Cancer Institute, which contain the latest treatment protocols for most cancers. These files are available elsewhere on CompuServe (and via Grateful Med), but you can get them here without paying surcharges. There are also a host of miscellaneous files containing a wide range of useful information — for example, the names of drug company representatives you can contact about providing free medication to financially needy patients. (The name of that file is *drugfr.lst*.)

The Cancer Forum's message board is subdivided into twenty-three topic areas chosen by a team of medical specialists. It includes twelve *medical* topics on cancer types, organized primarily by regions or organs of the body, such as *breast*, *gynecological*, *prostate*, and *skin*. Other subsections cover nonclinical topics, such as *insurance*, *nutrition*, and *legal*. You can read messages in all areas or just those that interest you.

WHAT HAPPENS ON THE CANCER FORUM

One evening the following message appeared in the breast cancer section of the Cancer Forum:

"My wife said, 'I found a lump in my breast.' . . . I feel numb right now. What do I do?"

Within a few hours, the worried husband received three responses — one of them from a physician. All three writers, after reminding him that most breast lumps prove to be benign cysts, agreed that this one called for an immediate medical exam because his message had mentioned a history of breast cancer in his wife's family. They suggested further reading, starting with files in the CompuServe Cancer Forum library.

"It's going to be kind of scary to read about this stuff," one correspondent warned, "but it's good to be prepared in case you have to make decisions. Ask the doctors as many questions as you can and ask questions here. There are a lot of breast cancer survivors on this forum as well as medical professionals."

Over the next few days the "I Have a Lump . . ." message thread grew longer and more personal. Former cancer patients wrote to offer both concrete advice and warm words of encouragement. Doctors expressed readiness to help interpret diagnoses and treatment options if the lump proved malignant.

A week later, thanking respondents for their support and advice, the man whose note began the thread joked that his tears might short out his keyboard. Within two more weeks, he was leaving his own advice for others on how to locate online information about breast cancer.

That's one fairly typical pattern of query and response.

"I see the process unfold," says Joanne Goldberg, a successful Cancer Forum searcher and frequent mentor to newcomers. "People come in with a question. Then the light dawns. It goes from 'Does anyone know anything about this?' to someone understanding her options."

ONLINE DISCUSSION GROUPS AFFIRM ACTIVE PATIENTS

Understanding your options is what participation in an online discussion group is all about. The people who participate almost certainly aren't a random sample of the population. It's far more likely that they're more active, better educated, and more inclined to ask questions than most people. Sometimes they engage in sharp debates.

One such debate involved the contention of Patient Advocates for Advanced Cancer Treatments (PAACT) that *all* prostate cancer therapies should be classified as "experimental" on the grounds that their relative merits have been insufficiently researched. A urologist (and regular participant in the prostate cancer section of the forum) complained, "The only thing that a new patient with questions gets here is a referral to PAACT and a reaffirmation that all of their positions are gospel. . . ." This elicited a rejoinder from another physician, also a regular participant, who contended that the forum generally, and PAACT in particular, provided a useful antidote to medical complacency about "standard" practices.

A number of patients chimed in. Most made a point of saying that they valued both doctors' participation in the forum and that they used PAACT literature not as "gospel" but as a starting point for identifying options their physicians often failed to mention. One patient summed up several messages as follows:

> I think the real lesson here is that there is no alternative but to involve patients in decisions about their care — I mean, really involve them. After all, when you are dealing with prostate cancer patients you are dealing with mature men. We have made decisions for our families for many years. Many of us have made decisions for small businesses or large organizations that involve many people and large sums of money. That crestfallen grown man slumped in a chair before the doctor, moments after he has been clobbered with a cancer diagnosis, is not a child.

Late in 1994 a similar but even stormier controversy erupted in the Cancer Forum over the message management policies of OncoLink, an Internet information clearinghouse providing both reference materials on cancer and a vehicle for exchanging questions and answers among patients and between patients and participating physicians. OncoLink was founded by Loren Buhle, Ph.D., an assistant professor of medical physics in radiation oncology at the University of Pennsylvania medical school, after his then three-year-old daughter was diagnosed with leukemia. OncoLink grew rapidly, to the point of receiving approximately ten thousand calls per day. Ultimately, physicians on the medical school staff insisted that Buhle cease posting materials (mostly nontechnical summaries of medical literature) that had not been approved by a medical doctor. They issued a statement that said "we all must recognize the harm which may be caused by distributing potentially erroneous, unconfirmed or unbalanced information to cancer patients and their families." Within days, more than fifty messages appeared on the Cancer Forum, mostly supporting Buhle and taking strong exception to the notion that patients should be protected by doctors from exposure to possible sources of error. The physicians prevailed. (OncoLink remains on the Internet as a less open but still useful resource.)

Controversies like these should not deter you from making full use of online message centers. They serve as a reminder that materials on online message centers may or may not undergo the kind of medical scrutiny associated with professional journals. Those who post messages on them, patients and physicians alike, can make mistakes or extrapolate inappropriately from their own experience. The strength of most online forums is their openness to give-and-take among participants and clarity in identifying the sources of posted information. Used uncritically, they can, like anything else, be dangerous; used intelligently, they are an invaluable asset in your search for medical information.

OTHER ONLINE MESSAGE CENTERS

Other medical message centers on CompuServe include the Diabetes Forum, the Disabilities Forum, and the Health and Fitness Forum, whose topical subsections include mental health and substance abuse. You should know about the American Medical Informatics Forum, which you reach by typing Go MEDSIG. Its sections focus on the kinds of problems that concern hospital administrators and academic researchers, such as quantitative measures of the quality of medical services, statistical validity of clinical trials data, and innovative uses of computers in medicine. From time to time, however, its members will respond to questions from patients on how to interpret technical or scientific material.

You will also find medical message centers on America Online, DELPHI, GEnie, and Prodigy. They tend to be less specialized than those on CompuServe, but participants are no less open and helpful.

Your best resource for locating direct-dial BBSs is the free Black Bag guide to medical lists, which provides names, phone numbers, and subject-matter descriptors (for example, AIDS, CANCER, PSYCH) for approximately four hundred other medical BBSs. These BBSs are free, but using them can run up substantial long-distance telephone charges. You can download this file from the Black Bag at (610) 454-7396 or from libraries within both the MEDSIG and CANCER forums on CompuServe.

INTERNET MAILING LISTS

Message centers abound on the Internet, where they are known as "Usenet groups," "Listserv discussion groups," or simply "lists." For example, there are more than three hundred *listserv* groups related to health and medical topics. By whatever name, they are functionally similar to CompuServe and other topic-oriented online forums. You can join many of these lists *without having full Internet access* by subscribing to a commercial online vendor. You can also find more than seventy Internet lists "echoed" on the Black Bag.

Basically, you join a list by sending an e-mail message to that list's Internet *listserv* address. *Listserv* is a computer program that maintains a discussion group subscription list and handles the mechanics of message transmission. The form of the e-mail address is usually *listserv@code-name-of-host-computer.institution-where-host-computer-is-located."domain"-of-institution.* For example, in the e-mail address *listserv@vm.temple.edu,* "vm" is the code name of the "host" computer where the list is maintained; the computer is located at Temple University in Philadelphia; and "edu" is a three letter "domain" code that in this case signifies an educational institution. (Occasionally, the form of the address will vary. *Listserv* is the most common program, but others perform similar functions in slightly different ways. The four most common, after listserv, are *Listproc, Mailserv, Mailbase,* and *Majordomo.*)

You can practice participation in Internet *listserv* groups by joining HELP-NET. To do this, you send a message to *listserv@vm.temple.edu.* The message you send should read as follows: *subscribe HELP-NET your-first-name your-last-name* (for example, *subscribe HELP-NET Jane Smith*). Usually within a few hours, you'll receive a "welcome to the list" message, along with some instructions on its rules and how to take advantage of anything special it offers, such as access to files. When and if you decide that HELP-NET no longer meets your needs, you send the message *unsubscribe HELP-NET*, again followed by your first and last names. If you want to stop mail temporarily — during a vacation, for example — the command is *set HELP-NET nomail;* to resume delivery, the command is *set HELP-NET mail.* You'll follow an identical procedure for any other *listserv* discussion group, sending your command message to that group's address and, of course, substituting that group's name for HELP-NET in the examples.

You can search for *listservs* on a particular topic by e-mail. If, for example, you wanted to find out what *listservs* exist on "aging," you might send the following message:

    To: listserv@american.edu
    Subject: [leave blank]
    list global /aging
    list global /geront
    list global /geriat.

That is, you list one search word, or part word, per line. (Note that the search function looks for a string of letters, so "aging" may also bring up lists that include such words as "managing" and "packaging.")

Usenet groups are similar in function and have different names, reflecting how they came into existence. You can locate Usenet groups with a gopher (a tool described in the following chapter) and reach them by e-mail with a process similar to posting *listserv* messages, described in detail in books on the Internet.

Internet lists are said to be "owned" by the individual or group that maintains them, and their rules vary. Many Internet lists are "open," meaning that anyone can join simply by following the procedure already described. Others are "closed," meaning that you must send the owner of the list a message explaining why you have a legitimate reason for participating. Examples of closed lists are those maintained solely for the benefit of members of a professional society and those that deal with child abuse, rape, and other sensitive issues where participants' privacy is extremely important. Also, some lists are "moderated" and others "unmoderated." In a moderated list, the owner or a designee retains the option of playing a role similar to that of a discussion leader, deciding which messages will be of interest to all participants and which are better handled by private e-mail between individual participants. They also decide which messages should go into archived "threads"; that is, into collections of messages on a single topic that, taken together, grow into something like conference transcripts.

A SAMPLE OF HEALTH-RELATED INTERNET LISTS

The number of Internet lists tends to grow by a kind of natural process, something like cell division. A particular list on, say, "cancer" will attract more and more members, many of whom are interested in a particular type of cancer. When enough people join the list who are mainly interested in, for example, breast cancer, one of them is likely to form a new list focusing on that disease. By the time you read this, there may be an Internet list dealing specifically with *male* breast cancer.

You can find health-related Internet lists in a guide to Internet resources called "The Medical List," compiled by Gary Malet, M.D., and Lee Hancock, an education technologist at the University of Kansas. This guide, cataloging Internet information sources, is described in more detail in chapter 13. The following sample of lists, adapted from Malet's and Hancock's work, provides some indication of the range of topics covered. If you don't see a list that interests you, one may nevertheless exist. (Bear in mind that Internet addresses change often, sometimes for technical reasons and sometimes because a list's sponsor changes.)

AIDSNews

The AIDSNews Forum is used for discussion of any issue related to AIDS and AIDS-related diseases. It reports on experimental and alternative treatments, especially those available now. It collects information from medical journals, interviews with scientists, physicians, and patients. It does not recommend therapies but seeks to increase participants' understanding of their options. It also distributes other publications, such as *AIDS Treatment News* and *Northern Lights Alternatives*. Subscribers' e-mail addresses are kept confidential to protect privacy. Address: *listserv@rutgers.edu*.

ALZHEIMER

This is an e-mail discussion group from patients, researchers, and caregivers (both family and professional) with an interest in Alzheimer's or related disorders in older adults. It provides an opportunity to exchange questions and answers both on the disease itself and on ways of coping with its effects. Address: *major-domo@wubios.wustl.edu*.

BMT-TALK

This is a list developed and moderated by Laurel Simmons, whose struggle with leukemia is described in chapter 2. It provides information on bone marrow transplants. Address: *bmt-talk@ai.mit.edu*.

BREASTCANCER

This is an open, unmoderated discussion list for researchers, physicians, patients, and families. This list is intended not only to provide for the exchange of therapeutic information but, to quote Malet and Hancock, "for the discussion of the work of various grassroots breast cancer advocacy groups worldwide . . . and, more broadly, to discuss the politics of breast cancer and health care." Address: *listserver@morgan.ucs.mun.ca*. Another cancer-oriented discussion group, not confined to a particular type of cancer, may be found at the following address: *listserv@wvnvn.wvnet*.

DIABETIC

This list is primarily for diabetic patients. Address: *listserv%pc-cvm.bitnet@cmsa.berkeley.edu*. (The extra symbols up front mean that this list is on a network called BITNET. If you were connecting from within the BITNET system, your local system manager would provide the exact address, which would be shorter than this one.) There's another list on diabetes, primarily for researchers. Its address is *listserv%irlearn.bitnet@hearn.nic.surfnet.nl*.

CARDIAC-PREV-

This Canadian list is open for discussion and questions on non-pharmacological prevention of coronary heart disease, such as attention to diet, exercise, and avoidance of smoking. Address: *mailserv@ac.dal.ca.*

IBDLIST

This is a moderated list discussing all aspects of inflammatory bowel diseases, with particular emphasis on Crohn's disease and ulcerative colitis. Address: *ibdlist-request%mvac23@udel.edu.*

GERINET

This is a list for those interested in geriatric health care, primarily professionals such as physicians, social workers, physical therapists, psychologists, and nursing home administrators. Address: *listserv@ubvm.cc.buffalo.edu.*

MENOPAUS

This is an open list, primarily for sharing personal experiences related to menopause. Some physicians participate. Address: *listserv@psuhmc.maricopa.edu.*

WITSENDO

This is a moderated list for discussing all aspects of endometriosis. Address: *listserv@dartcms1.dartmouth.edu.*

CFS-L

This is an open, unmoderated list for persons with chronic fatigue syndrome (CFS), characterized by debilitating fatigue and flu-like symptoms. Address: *listserv@list.nih.gov.*

IMMUNE

This list is for discussion of problems associated with chronic fatigue, lupus, or allergies relating to immune system breakdowns. Address: *listserv@weber.ucsd.edu.*

BRAINTMR

This is a brain tumor forum, in which both patients and researchers participate actively. Address: *listserv@mitmvma.mit.edu.*

DOWN-SYN

This is a listserv mailing list for discussion of Down's syndrome. Address: *listserv@vm1.nodak.edu.*

PARKINSN

Topics related to Parkinson's disease are discussed here. Address: *listserv@vm.utcc.utoronto.ca.*

STROKE-L

This is for stroke-related topics. Address: *listserv@ukcc.uky.edu.*

BACKS-L

This is for those doing research on, and treatment of, lower back pain, disability, and rehabilitation. Address: *listserv@moose.uv.edu.*

SOREHAND

This list deals with carpal tunnel syndrome, tendinitis, and similar problems. Address: *listserv@ubvm.cc.buffalo.edu.*

CYSTIC FIBROSIS

This is a private list whose Internet address is *listserv-@frmop11.cnusc.fr.* (The *fr* in the "domain" part of the address means that the host computer is in France.) For more details, contact *jorda@frsun12*.

SCHIZOPH

Participants include professionals, individuals, and family members who are concerned with schizophrenia. Internet address: *listserv@vm.utcc.utoronto.ca*.

TRAUMATIC-STRESS

This is for persons interested in the study and treatment of the consequences of highly stressful events. Address: *mailbase@mailbase.ac.uk*. (The "uk" means that the owner of the list is in the United Kingdom — that is, Great Britain.) For more information, contact *cfigley@garnet.acns.fsu.edu*.

TRNSPLNT

This is an independent discussion forum for organ transplant recipients. The list's owner identifies himself as the recipient of kidney transplants. Address: *danf___cm@wuvmd.wustl.edu*.

A LITTLE BIT OF LURKING

Once on a list, you do not have to do anything in particular to remain a member. A high percentage of participants are "lurkers," a term that carries no negative implications. That is, lurkers read messages but seldom write them.

If you lurk on a list, you're reading someone's mail — with that person's permission. Some messages may be instantly clear. ("It's hard to describe the effects — some chills and fever but mainly just this nauseous feeling and general malaise.") Others may be cryptic, understandable only by physicians and a handful of patients. ("Are you sure about the dosage? . . . I also get Intron A 5 mio. I.U. daily to keep my CML in chronic phase.")

Mostly, you can expect to pick up contacts and ideas.

Consider the following excerpts from an Internet discussion group on chronic fatigue syndrome (CFS). A participant named Bill writes that he's often too tired even to sit up and read. Someone named Carol advises him to order "Talking Books" from the Library of Congress:

> *Carol:* . . . All free. They sent me a special cassette player and all the tapes I want. The selection is amazing. Now, all those hours I have to spend lying on the bed with my eyes closed are spent listening to books and getting well-read.
>
> *Bill:* You mean CFS qualifies one for this service? I thought it was only for visually impaired folks.
>
> *Carol:* I think it used to be for the blind, but it's now for the blind and handicapped. You do need your doctor's signature. Happy reading!
>
> *A new participant named Susan adds to the thread*: Talking Books are for ANYONE with special needs — back problems, broken arms, pregnancy, you name it — as long as your doctor is willing to sign off on the excuse.

The exchange of information here may not be as dramatic as news of a wonder drug, but it's useful to someone facing an extended period of being bedridden much of the day. It's an example of information you won't find on MEDLINE or that you can scarcely expect your doctor to remember to mention, even if he or she knows it.

TIPS ON EFFECTIVE NETWORKING

In any message center environment — a commercial vendor's forum, a private BBS, or the Internet — making effective use of the resource is mostly a matter of common sense and courtesy. Here are a few suggestions:

- Pay attention to how you label your message. The heading you choose will be the only part of your message that many readers scanning the BBS will read. Your label will normally be limited to a small number of characters. Anyone scanning the Cancer Forum message titles instantly understands "I Have a Lump . . ." as a call for help. Usually, however, your label should be as specific as space permits. "Stage 4 Colon Chemo??" is more likely to attract an appropriate specialist than "Patient Needs Advice."
- Make your message itself as specific as possible. If you're asking for advice on treatment, mention what's already been tried. For example, the following paragraph introduced a message on the Cancer Forum:

> ["Jane Doe"] is a 31 year old woman, whose diagnosis is stage IV recurrent breast carcinoma with secondary brain metastasis; she has had both a right and left modified radical mastectomy. She has been treated with regular protocols of adjuvant chemotherapy, external electron beam radiation with varying intensities, hyperthermia, single agent chemotherapy and brain irradiation. . . .

Not surprisingly, the request for advice that followed elicited equally specific responses. Moreover, one is far more likely to get a constructive private message from this kind of posting than from one that is general or vague.

- Stick to the subject. Adding a few lines of personal information is OK and may even help readers relate to you more easily, but people don't read a prostate cancer board for your opinions on national health care reform.
- If you respond to a question, reply with a public posting only on matters of general interest or with answers from which others might benefit. Otherwise, reply directly to the individual. (On the Internet, a public message is called a message "to the list." If you get a number of private answers to a question that may be of general interest, such as the usefulness of some database, it's courteous to summarize answers in one public posting to the list.)

• Don't forget that you can send participants private messages. For example, if you're monitoring an Internet mail list used by neurosurgeons, you may want to send a personal e-mail note (with an appropriately polite introduction) to a specialist who you think can answer a specific technical question.

• When posting questions on boards for professionals (and certainly when contacting individual professionals), be considerate of their time and recognize that their responses to questions reflect courtesy and a sense of public service, not obligation. Inconsiderate questioning can jeopardize everyone's access to expertise by causing a professional board to exclude outsiders.

• Help someone else whenever you can. Online message centers work only because many people, from highly trained professionals to individuals whose insights were acquired through personal suffering, share whatever knowledge or expertise they possess. The way you pay them back is by sharing whatever you can whenever you're able to do so.

A Few Things to Watch Out For

You really have little to lose by at least scanning online message centers as part of your search for the best treatment. Nevertheless, here are a few cautions:

• Maintain your objectivity about the advice you receive. If your doctor has been uncommunicative, it can be so refreshing to hear from people who are intelligent, eager to help, and apparently well informed that it's easy to forget that they, too, are fallible. Online discussion groups facilitate your search for information; they're no substitute for carefully researched medical advice.

• Subscribing to an Internet discussion group can be like drinking from a fire hose. On some lists, you may receive between twenty and fifty messages per day. That kind of sudden information surge is more than disconcerting; it can be expensive if you get your mail through a commercial service that charges for incoming messages. So try out no more than a very few lists at a time, and be sure to save the instructions you'll be given on the first day about how to get *off* an Internet mailing list. (As noted earlier, the usual command is *unsubscribe*, followed by your name. On some lists the command is *signoff*.)

• Technical glitches happen, especially on the Internet. Sometimes you can have trouble signing on to a mailing list for no obvious reason. Who knows why? The Internet addresses listed in this chapter are easy to type incorrectly. Check to see if an address is case-sensitive and if you typed a lowercase letter when you should have typed a capital letter. Maybe you made some other slip of the fingers, like typing an "l" (ell) when you should have typed a "1" (one), or a "u" for a "v." Maybe you did nothing wrong, but some problem occurred during transmission or with the host computer. (Computers at high-traffic places like major universities do fall behind, and sometimes they go down.) Maybe the address has changed. If you're unsuccessful after several tries, post a question describing your problem on a related message center. Networking is not an exact science, but you can usually find the resource you need if you ask around.

• In cyberspace, as elsewhere, you may now and then be treated discourteously. Sometimes an innocent question will elicit a sharp rebuke, or "flame" message. Apologize if you feel you made a mistake; otherwise, ignore it. Happily, flaming is rare on medical and patient-centered message lists.

• If you download a program (such as one intended to help you locate, organize, or display data), use a commercial antivirus program to check it out before running it in your computer. Fortunately, there is no known way for you to contract a computer virus merely by reading an e-mail message.

COMPUTERS AND HUMAN CONTACTS

Many of the people whose stories have been told in this book — Valerie Brown, Joanne Goldberg, Al Musella, Valerie Ostroth, Ronald Surface — are regular participants in one or more online discussion groups. Some are active searchers for medical information on their own behalf; some are mentors for patients new to online services. Most of them are a bit of both.

You may occasionally hear someone say, "I'm not comfortable with computers; I like *human* contact." In fact, human contact is what online message centers are all about. Whether they are called "forums," "discussion groups," or "lists," their function is to widen your range of human contacts and reinforce a sense of community.

What Ostroth, speaking of her online activities, said of persons with CFS/CFIDS tends to be true of any seriously ill person: "My social contact has dropped significantly since I became ill. We are often so alienated or alone that the human contact is vital for the survival of our minds."

She and others make several points. People are often less self-conscious in typing onscreen messages than they would be in person, or even on the telephone. Individuals with illnesses that make it difficult or impossible for them to travel can participate in group activities without going to meetings. Patients can enter and read messages at any hour of the day or night, whenever their energy level permits. Surface calls computers "the ultimate form of handicapped access."

Valerie Brown, whose online searches helped her husband, Mike, to "fight like hell," comments that without online coaching from fellow searchers, she "would have never known where to start" in thinking through specific issues. She adds:

> When you go through a serious illness like this, you don't know what questions to ask. For example, there's a lady on the forum whose husband had been through it twice. She suggested that we get copies of every single medical report they did on Mike because when we went to seek a second opinion we would have all the information right with us and wouldn't have to track it down. This is something that only someone who's been through it would have come up with.

Valerie spent a week working up her courage before logging on to the Cancer Forum. Now she says:

> It makes me feel good now to be able to post a message to somebody and say, "It's going to be OK. I know what you're going through and there's good days and there's bad." Maybe what I say doesn't really help, but I think it does because of people that responded to me when *I* needed it.

13.

Medical Resources on the Internet

THE INTERNET HAS been both over-hyped and over-mystified. As a phenomenon, it's every bit as amazing as the popular press makes it sound, but it's not always as useful for the average medical information searcher as commercial services that organize data for the convenience of paying customers. But you don't have to be a computer wizard to learn to search it. In fact, distinctions between the Internet and commercial services are blurring because providers like America Online, CompuServe, and Prodigy are competing to offer easy Internet access.

The Internet is the sum of over twenty thousand computer-based networks that connect many millions of individual users. It's growing incredibly fast and and changing as it grows. It's like a huge city, or a small nation, in which people go about their own business and pursue their own interests. Many of its addresses are strictly for business or private communication, not for tourists. Others are public, open to anyone at any hour.

The Internet provides a pathway to many medical resources, both databases and ways of contacting knowledgeable people.

Some of these are available *only* via the Internet. Others are available less expensively on the Internet than elsewhere.

This chapter does *not* attempt to provide detailed instructions on doing Internet searches. That would require far too much space and duplicate existing books on the Internet. There are scores of books on the Internet in print, and more are appearing all the time. (*The Internet Navigator*, by Paul Gilster, is especially comprehensive and readable.) Moreover, because the number of people beginning to use the Internet is creating a demand for easier ways to access it, you may not need to learn a lot of the search protocols of the kind mentioned in this chapter and still common on many institutional systems. New search tools are being developed at an extremely rapid rate, both by regular Internet users and by commercial access providers. In short, the Internet is in the process of changing from an environment dominated by scientists, computer experts, and university-based academics to an environment in which those knowledge professionals are joined by millions of people without special training in computers or online searching.

HOW TO CONNECT TO THE NET

If you've ever sent an e-mail message from CompuServe to someone at America Online, or vice versa, you've used the Internet as the pathway between the two systems. E-mail is the most basic and least demanding level of Internet access, and all of the commercial online services offer it. Usually, however, they add a charge for messages to addresses outside their own systems.

Full Internet access, however, includes access to the tools to search a wide range of databases and to participate in discussion groups. This requires either access to an institutional account or a subscription to a commercial online service offering Internet access. Much of the information on the Internet is free, but access to the system itself isn't — and never has been. Until recently, Internet connections were designed for purchase by universities and other employers for a flat monthly or annual fee, which enabled them to provide unlimited access to faculty, students, or staff.

Now you can buy access from many commercial vendors catering to small businesses and individuals, including the major online services. DELPHI was the first of the major commercial vendors to provide full, or nearly full, Internet access, but the others have largely caught up. Most also have online forums dedicated to Internet issues to enable members to ask questions, share experiences, and post search tips. Some also add surcharges for Internet access other than simple e-mail.

A great many local and regional services, mostly in urban areas, specialize in providing Internet access. Their advantage over the national vendors is that they may offer you local-call access at very high modem speeds, which are a near-necessity for downloading really long text files and most graphics files. But you must pay long-distance telephone charges if you live outside a regional vendor's immediate service area. In compensation, some of these vendors provide communications software that makes Internet searches relatively easy.

The best place to locate up-to-date information on regional options for connecting to the Internet is on the Internet itself. That's not a Catch-22 situation, since you can get a current list of regional vendors from the Public Dialup Internet Access List by sending an e-mail message from any commercial online service to *info-deli-server@netcom.com*. The message should read *send PDIAL*. The list is free, but your online vendor will charge for its own equivalent of postage and handling. PDIAL is a file several pages long, so a vendor's transmission surcharges won't bankrupt you, but some Internet files are as long as small books and can take several hundred pages to print out. At modem speeds below 9600 baud they can take the better part of an hour to download. It can be *very* expensive to receive files of this size via commercial services.

THE TOOLS OF INTERNET SEARCHES

From an information searcher's point of view, the main problem with the Internet is that it contains too much information, scattered across too many locations. Its thousands of interconnected networks (that's thousands of *networks*, remember, not merely thousands of computers) comprise a mega-network so vast and containing so many files that searching it without specialized tools would be like trying to find a single phone number in a metropolitan telephone directory that no one had bothered to alphabetize.

This section will give only the briefest of introductions to Internet search tools, just enough to clarify a few necessary references later. The tools themselves aren't hard to use; the difficulty lies in knowing which tool is needed in what situation. If you work for an institution with Internet access, someone in your computer department will already have loaded most of these tools into the institution's computer. If you're operating from your home, you may wish to consult Gilster's *The Internet Navigator* or perhaps order *Internet for Medical Librarians: A Syllabus* by Dudee Chiang, a librarian at the University of Southern California. Soon you may not even need a book. Increasingly, these tools are being built into software provided by commercial vendors who provide Internet access for a fee. For the present, however, at least some knowledge of the Internet tool kit remains useful.

E-mail

It may seem odd to refer to e-mail as a *tool*. It's mentioned here because you can sign on to many of the Internet discussion lists simply by sending an e-mail message to the list's owner. The usual message form is *subscribe name of list your name*. Do not add extra questions or messages like "thanks in advance."

Telnet

Telnet provides you with a way of connecting to a remote computer, known as a "host" computer, in order to perform some function, like search a database. The host may be across town from you or across the country. For example, to search the MEDLARS family of databases (which includes MEDLINE) at the National Library of Medicine, you would begin by typing *telnet medlars.nlm.nih.gov*. (As already noted, you'd need an account before you could actually do the search.) You'll often see *telnet* used as a verb, as in "To reach MEDLINE, first telnet to *medlars.nlm.nih.gov.*"

FTP

FTP stands for *file transfer protocol.* It's the principal Internet tool for transferring files from one computer to another. Many computer databases contain sensitive information (for example, personnel and payroll data) and are closed to outside searchers. However, many institutions reserve certain areas of computer memory for public access by way of "anonymous ftp." When prompted for your name by these "FTP sites," you type in "anonymous" and use your Internet address as your password. Once you reach the computer where the data you want is stored, you'll need to know a few other commands to locate and download the file you want, but they're simple and usually intuitive, like "dir" (for directory), "get," and "quit."

Gopher

FTP is easy to use once you know the address where the information you want is located, but it can't help you find that address. A *gopher* helps you find it. It's a sort of electronic table of contents for cross-referenced areas of the Internet.

Gophers organize Internet information in a hierarchical order and display the contents of databases in a series of menus. The databases need not be at the same site. For example, the National Library of Medicine has a gopher, and Figure 13-1 shows some of the information its opening menu displays, followed by what you'd see on a second screen if you asked for more information on the entry "NLM Publications." Selecting the entry "Other Gophers" would lead you to other computers.

Within the Internet, you reach the NLM's gopher by typing *gopher gopher.nlm.nih.gov* unless you have a graphically oriented communications program that permits you to point and click with a mouse.

Individually, gophers are programs located within the computer system from which you are searching. However, they con-

---

[First menu page]

1. About this gopher (which is still under construction).
2. About the National Library of Medicine.
3. NLM Publications . . . /
4. NLM Online Services . . . /
5. Other Gophers . . . /

[A second-level menu page]

1. Files add/updated in last 30 days (since [date]) . . . /
2. AIDS Publications . . . /
3. Current Bibliographies in Medicine . . . /
4. Information about the Unified Medical Language System . . . /
   [etc.]

Figure 13-1a. Menus from National Library of Medicine gopher.

nect with each other to comprise a logical area that Internet searchers often call "gopherspace," so that when you've reached one gopher you've virtually reached them all. Gophers provide access to far more types of information than FTP, which only allows you to retrieve files. Each gopher was once designed by some programmer to assist a particular kind of research, and the logic of that research may not be quite the same as yours. Nevertheless, gophers are a helpful and easy-to-use tool.

Archie

Archie derives from "archive." It refers to a program that enables a keyword search of directories at many different FTP sites containing files downloadable by *anonymous ftp* (explained above under "FTP"). If your computer doesn't have an *archie client*, meaning a program that performs this search function, you can *telnet* (remotely connect) to a computer that does have one.

NLM Gopher

File   Edit   Options   Bookmarks   Recent   Help

NLM Gopher information. searching and new files

NLM Fact Sheets, Newsletters, Reports, Agreements and Forms

AIDS information

Extramural Programs (Grants and Contracts)

Grateful Med

HSTAT – Health Services/Technology Assessment Texts

National Institutes of Health (NIH) Clinical Alerts

Online services

Resource lists and bibliographies

Technical services resources and information

Toxicology and Environmental Health Information Program

Unified Medical Language System (UMLS) information

Visible Human Project

NLM Staff Information (Internal)

Tunnels to other gophers

BCGopher(tm) ©1993, 1994 Boston College

Figure 13-1b. Menu from National Library of Medicine gopher.

File Edit Options Bookmarks Recent   Help

Gratefully Yours

Grateful Med Fact Sheet [7Oct94 8K]

[PS] Grateful Med Fact Sheet [29Sep94 748K]

Loansome Doc Fact Sheet [26Aug94 6K]

[PS] Loansome Doc Fact Sheet [17Aug94 178K]

Order form for Grateful Med [4May94 2K]

Application for MEDLARS User ID. Required for Grateful Med. [4May94 12K]

BCGopher™ ©1993, 1994 Boston College

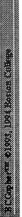

Figure 13-1c. Menu from National Library of Medicine gopher.

Veronica

Veronica is a program built into many but not all individual gophers that permits a keyword search of all gopher menus to which a gopher you have reached is connected — that is, of "gopherspace." It resembles *archie*, except that it searches gopher menus rather than the contents of a particular computer network, and, unlike *archie*, it enables you to eliminate a separate ftp session to retrieve the file.

World Wide Web

The *World Wide Web* (WWW) is a program that lets you search the Internet in many different ways, beginning anywhere you like — with a topic like "medicine" or a tool like "WHOIS" (an Internet address searcher). You can move back and forth across categories with ease, from a subtopic under "medicine" to something related to one of those subtopics that is also reachable under "economics," "law," or maybe even "religion." It's based on a powerful search tool called *hypertext* and lets you follow your own interests or intuition. With hypertext, keywords in the text on your computer screen are highlighted. If you select a highlighted word, you are immediately routed to a source containing information regarding that word. Frequently, that source is at another site, perhaps in another part of the world. Although the Web is searchable by text commands, the use of icon-based software known as "Web browsers" has become almost universal. You can use a Web browser provided by the vendor from whom you purchase your Internet connection, or buy a separate product. Web sites (addresses) are likely to offer colorful graphics, but graphics require transmitting lots of data, so you need a high-speed modem (at least 14,400 baud) for effective Web searches.

World Wide Web addresses for medical resources (whose indexes are called "home pages") are multiplying on the Internet with amazing rapidity. Almost any issue of "Medical Matrix News," an online newsletter described below, lists a dozen new ones. A glossary of Internet terms may be found at the following address: http://www.matisse.net/files/glossary.html.

In summary, some Internet search tools have nearly universal utility, and others work only in certain environments. Almost any form of direct Internet access will give you all the tools you need for text searches, though not for sound and graphics.

As already noted, commercial vendors are scrambling to make Internet access easier. The future of Internet searching seems to lie with WWW or hypertext tools, known generically as "Web browsers." *Mosaic* is one example. Commercial packages include names like "NetCruiser" and "Internet in a Box." The commercial packages typically incorporate tools like *archie* and *gopher*, but you don't type in those commands. Instead, you use a computer mouse to point and click on screen icons. Finally, communication giants like MCI, whose telephone networks carry 40 percent of Internet traffic, and AT&T are entering the competition to provide direct Internet access to nontechnical customers.

WHAT YOU CAN FIND ON THE INTERNET — AN OVERVIEW

As with online medical resources already discussed, it is convenient to consider Internet resources under two broad headings: reference materials (in databases and publications) and people (in discussion groups and e-mail lists). Of course, as explained in previous chapters, you often find reference materials and knowledgeable people at the same addresses, just as libraries have both books and places for patrons to read and talk.

The category *reference materials* may in turn be divided into *interactive databases* and *files*. Generally speaking, you will *not* want to use the Internet for searching interactive databases like MEDLINE, because it's not as easy as other methods. Of course, if you have free access to the Internet through your employer, then you may want to use that system for interactive searches. You'll still need a MEDLINE account. That is, even if Internet access is free to you, there'll still be a charge for the MEDLINE search itself. If you don't have free access, Grateful Med's one-time cost of about $30 is a better bargain.

The Internet abounds in medical *files* that you can download to your computer but cannot search through interactively as you can with MEDLINE. Many, perhaps most, of these files are free for the taking if you know how to find them. Yet many of those most in demand are available elsewhere — in CompuServe forum libraries and on direct-dial bulletin boards. The reason is simple. The people who maintain or make regular use of online services and medical BBSs transfer what they think will interest others to their own libraries. So you often have a choice: searching the scattered libraries of the Internet for information that's free (once you've paid a flat fee for access) or paying a bit more in online time charges for the convenience of an online shopping mall like CompuServe.

The best reason for Internet access is access to people, especially experts. As noted in the previous chapter, Internet discussion groups (whether on BITNET networks or elsewhere) tend to be developed by and for specialists. They're busy professionals, but if you approach them with specific questions you'll usually get helpful answers. ("I've searched MEDLINE but haven't found anything that directly compares the risks and benefits of cryosurgery vs. a radical prostatectomy. . . .")

LOCATING INTERNET MEDICAL RESOURCES

The most comprehensive job of mapping the medical resources available on the Internet has been done by Gary Malet, M.D., and Lee Hancock, an education technologist at the University of Kansas. They have compiled a guide to online medical information known as "The Internet Health Science Resources List." (A subset of this list, known simply as "The Medical List," includes only sources of clinical information.) The most recent full-length version of the list prints out at over four hundred single-spaced pages. It is copyrighted but available without charge via the Internet. The command sequence is as follows (prompts are shown in italics and comments in brackets):

ftp ftp2.cc.ukans.edu
Login: anonymous [lowercase necessary]
Password: [your e-mail address]

cd [for "change directory"] pub/hmatrix
get medlst03.txt [or a later number than "03"]
Transfer complete
quit

More detailed instructions are available by e-mail from *gmalet@surfer.win.net*. The list can also be downloaded from the MEDSIG forum on CompuServe. (Do remember that downloading a file this size is costly.) For Internet users able to do World Wide Web searches, "The Internet Health Science Resources List" has been entered in a format called *hypertext* that can facilitate online keyword searches from a home computer.

The lists of Internet resources in this and the preceding chapter represent only a fraction of the resources listed in Malet's and Hancock's list, which is regularly updated. (In January 1995 alone, more than seventy new groups were added.) If you decide that the Internet should be part of your search for the best treatment, download either version of the "Medical List" or find someone who'll copy one to a disk and mail it to you.

Malet and Hancock also edit an online periodic publication supported by the American Medical Infomatics Association Internet Working Group. It is called "Medical Matrix News" and lists a sample of new medical discussion groups on the Internet and reports on projects to facilitate Internet access. To receive it, send an e-mail message to *listproc@kumchttp.mc.ukans.edu* with the first line *subscribe mmatrix-L yourfirstname yourlastname*.

A SHORT INTERNET MEDICAL SAMPLER

The following section lists a few of the more important Internet information sources available to you — a mere handful out of a list of addresses numbered in the thousands. Please be aware that many Internet information resources are developed by individual faculty members or other researchers for noncommercial reasons. For that reason, *any* Internet address is more likely to change over the course of a few years than are the addresses of major commercial services.

MEDLINE

As mentioned, you can connect to MEDLINE via an Internet pathway, but you'll still need an account to do an actual search. If this option interests you, you're probably already associated with an institution that has Internet access, so your organization's librarian or computer center can help you make connections.

CANCERNET

This provides a way to obtain comprehensive and current cancer information from the National Cancer Institute (NCI). You can request information from the NCI's PDQ database, fact sheets on cancer topics, and abstracts from the CANCERLIT database, which includes cancer-related materials from MEDLINE. NCI does not charge for this service, but the vendor through which you acquire Internet access may charge for downloads. You can also, however, if you know what you want, simply call (800) 4CANCER to have material sent by surface mail or fax. The main advantage of online searching is the ability to browse through related materials.

To reach CANCERNET online, send e-mail to: *cancernet@icicb. nci.nih.gov* with no subject, and the word "help" as the message. You will get a message explaining how to use the system. CANCERNET can be searched with gopher, ftp, and World Wide Web. Much of its frequently requested material is also available in the protocols library of the CompuServe Cancer Forum.

CLINALRT

Clinical Alerts are announcements of interim clinical findings derived from research studies sponsored by the National Institutes of Health. These announcements are made prior to research reports in the peer-reviewed literature when the interim results are promising in reducing deaths or the effects of illness. To receive these alerts by e-mail, send the message *subscribe CLINALRT your- firstname yourlastname* to *listserv@umab.umd.edu.* You cannot screen by topic. For example, your concern may be limited to colon cancer, but you'll also get material on breast cancer, prostate cancer, and so on.

OncoLink

OncoLink is a well-organized source of cancer-related information maintained by the University of Pennsylvania School of Medicine. It contains a mixture of journal articles, more general reference materials, and newsletters on a wide range of cancer types and cancer-related issues. Its menus are divided into four general categories: (1) disease sites (for example, breast cancer, ovarian cancer); (2) medical specialties (for example, medical oncology, radiation oncology); (3) news items (for example, FDA/CDC announcements); and (4) links to other cancer-related resources on the Internet. During its first year of operation, it handled approximately 1,250,000 separate transactions.

OncoLink is accessible using either of two search tools, *gopher* or *World Wide Web*. Using a gopher, you type: *gopher cancer.med. upenn.edu 80*. Using a WWW-client, type: *http://cancer.med. upenn.edu/*.

PharmInfoNet

This is a WWW site for pharmaceutical information. It includes a database of articles, a list of frequently asked questions about drugs with answers from pharmaceutical manufacturers, a moderated archive of drug-related discussion threads, and links to other Internet sites of interest to pharmaceutical professionals. Its address is *URL:http://pharminfo.com*. For more information, send e-mail to *pialtd@ix.netcom.com* or call (800) 584-1063.

MEDNews Health Infocom Newsletter

This is an electronic newsletter, published weekly, containing health-related articles from around the world. Many of them are collected from government reports. The contents of this particular newsletter are more likely to interest health professionals than individuals searching for treatment options. Nevertheless, you may want to investigate it for yourself, because online newsletters may represent the wave of the future for communication among people with special interests, combining as they do rapid delivery with low publication and distribution costs.

To subscribe, send e-mail to *listserv@asuacad.bitnet* with the message line *subscribe MEDNEWS yourfirstname yourlastname.*

The newsletter is large and arrives in multiple sections, which facilitates its movement through the electronic network. If you decide it's not for you, promptly send the message *unsubscribe MEDNEWS yourfirstname yourlastname* to the same address.

LymeNet Newsletter

This is a specialized example of the same electronic publishing phenomenon. Subscribers to LymeNet-L receive the "LymeNet Newsletter" approximately twice a month. This publication provides readers with the latest research, treatment, and political news about Lyme disease. Contact Marc Gabriel, "LymeNet Newsletter," *mcg2@lehigh.edu.*

WMN-HLTH

Women's Health Electronic News Line. This is one more example of an electronic newsletter. The Internet address is *listserv@uwavm.u.-washington.edu.*

AS ALWAYS, THE DECISION IS YOURS

If you've already decided that you want Internet access but don't work for an organization that provides it, here are some suggestions.

• If you conclude that you need Internet access mainly for e-mail, you should stick with a commercial vendor. You can subscribe to discussion groups by e-mail, but you should be selective in this. Otherwise, you could find yourself running up quite a bill from handling charges on your increased mail volume.

• If you can get free access through an institutional account, it's worth the trouble of learning how to use what may at first seem a baffling system. (Telnet, gopher, and FTP, for example, are actually quite easy to use and will meet many of your needs. You don't have to learn everything at once.)

• The major commercial vendors are competing hard to provide full Internet access and may well represent the best choice for most users. The ease of access they provide justifies their charges.

• If you are a high-speed Internet user or if high-speed connections are important to you (perhaps for reasons unrelated to medical searches), unless you live in a very rural area, you can locate a local or regional vendor that specializes in providing full Internet access that permits such connections.

Even if you decide that you need full Internet access, including the ability to do WWW searches, you will probably find the conventional commercial vendors like America Online and CompuServe to be your best choice. The convenience they provide improves as they compete with each other for new customers who aren't experienced computer users. This convenience more than offsets their charges. Most national vendors even provide 800 numbers to enable customers in remote rural areas to avoid paying phone companies for toll calls, but the vendors do add their own surcharges for this service.

Ultimately, all that matters to you is your ability to access databases and online discussion groups, not whether or not you're doing that on something called "the Internet." Often you may neither know nor care where in cyberspace an information resource is located, except as it affects your cost of using it. (One exception occurs when you want to know where an expert lives or works because you plan to make offline contact by mail or telephone.)

In short, "surfing" the Internet is still not as easy as using the telephone and nowhere near as easy as surfing the channels on your television set. But competition is moving the system in that direction. Meanwhile, you might well base your decision on whether or how to connect to the Internet on whether you expect your searches to be relatively short and specific or part of a long, continuing process, as in the case of a chronic illness. From a long-term perspective, you'll sooner or later want access to the Internet and its search tools, especially since access is rapidly getting cheaper and the tools are becoming easier to use.

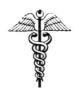

PART IV

YOU CAN COPE WITH

SPECIAL PROBLEMS

Finding the best treatment often involves more than locating information. You may need to learn abut participating in clinical trials, to consider the option of commissioning data searches, or to cope with insurance problems, which can be more troublesome than ever under managed health care. Even so, knowing your *medical* options remains your key to making effective decisions. As your skill in finding and analyzing information increases, so should your confidence in your own judgment.

14.

What You Need to Know about Clinical Trials

JUNE IN NEW ENGLAND can lift the spirit. Spring has done its good work, leaving behind the last traces of winter. But for Gary Schine, a June day in 1990 held a terrible poignancy: he learned from his doctor that he had an incurable leukemia.

As told in chapter 3, Gary did some research and found a promising new treatment that was being tested in a clinical trial. He was able to enroll in the study, which was being conducted in La Jolla, California, at the Scripps Clinic and Research Foundation, where the new agent (2-chlorodeoxyadenosine [2-CDA]) was developed. Gary spent seven days there receiving 2-CDA by intravenous infusion and another two weeks in posttreatment. Since that time, he has been free of his disease. The doctors tell him there's every reason to believe he will not suffer a relapse, and he has lived to see his young sons growing up.

NEW AVENUES FOR FINDING THE BEST TREATMENT

The preceding chapters primarily offer suggestions for finding information about treatment options sufficiently well studied to

212 ■ INFOMEDICINE

have been the subject of published articles. But what if your researches reveal nothing truly promising or if you are receiving a treatment that seems not to be working? In such circumstances, you may want to consider entering a clinical trial. Participation in a clinical trial may involve some risks, but it also gives you an opportunity to receive a new therapy that has not yet become part of the repertoire of standard clinical practice.

This chapter outlines the nature of clinical trials, how and why they are conducted, their advantages and drawbacks, and the specific conditions under which they may help patients looking for the best treatment.

WHAT ARE CLINICAL TRIALS?

Clinical trials are another name for clinical research formulated to study scientifically new medical treatments. Clinical trials *evaluate new therapies*, although trials may also involve the study of disease prevention, diagnosis, and detection, or the psychological impact of disease.

Most clinical trials are sponsored by the National Institutes of Health (NIH), the Veterans Administration (VA), or pharmaceutical companies — as single or joint efforts. Any drug or implanted device (such as a pacemaker) must be tested in clinical trials and deemed safe and effective on the basis of those trials before the Food and Drug Administration (FDA) will approve commercial use.

For a trial to be acceptable to the FDA, certain standard procedures are required. These include the establishment (normally by a steering committee) of a *study protocol* — a blueprint of a plan for the study. The protocol — usually a long, highly detailed document — states the scientific objectives of the trial, the strategy for carrying them out, and includes an exact treatment plan for patients.

Another requirement is that all trial enrollees must sign an informed consent document. Internationally agreed-upon guidelines for human experimentation, which are based upon the Nuremberg Code (1946) and the Declaration of Helsinki (1964), are grounded in the concept of voluntary consent. A doctor or trial coordinator must spell out every aspect of treatment: the type of drug or treatment being tested; how it will be administered; restrictions on any other drugs the patient is taking; hoped-for benefits; possible side effects, and the understanding that the patient can withdraw from participation any time. After the treatment protocol has been explained, patients willing to participate in the study must sign a release, also called an *informed consent form.*

An institution may not conduct a clinical trial without approval by an internal review board (IRB), sometimes called a clinical investigation committee (CIC). This is an independent group comprised of doctors, scientists, nurses, and community members. Its role is to appraise the study design (including treatment protocol) and monitor informed consent and patient safety.

TRIAL PROGRESSION

Clinical trials are carried out in three principal phases, with each stage designed to provide specific information:

Phase I

Phase I trials are the shortest of the three phases, lasting from a few days to one or two weeks. These studies are the first to take place outside the laboratory and with human subjects. Their purpose is to determine safe dosage levels and the best way of delivering the drug into a patient's system.

Participants are often healthy male volunteers and sometimes females of non-childbearing age. Toxic drugs, however, such as those used against cancer or AIDS, are never tested in healthy volunteers, but in patients who have the disease to be treated. Since participation in studies of toxic drugs may involve risks, these trials are mostly limited to patients who would not be helped with other known treatments.

Phase II

Phase II trials, utilizing larger numbers of participants (usually one hundred to four hundred), test how patients with the same disease respond to the drug being tested. This is the first phase primarily designed to test the effectiveness of a new drug or treatment on a significant scale. For example, patients with breast cancer not responding to standard therapy (i.e., their tumors fail to decrease in size) may be treated with a Phase II treatment. In addition to monitoring patients for response in a Phase II trial, investigators record and assess for the first time any side effects.

If a treatment is shown to be effective in a Phase II trial, it progresses to Phase III.

Phase III

Phase III trials are primarily designed to compare the effectiveness of a new therapy with that of a standard treatment. These trials require the participation of very large numbers of patients with the same disease, often divided randomly into two groups for scientific purposes: a control group, receiving standard treatment (or sometimes a placebo), and the second group, receiving the newly developed treatment or drug. These studies are conducted as "single-blind" or "double-blind" trials. In a single-blind trial, patients do not know which treatment they are receiving; in a double-blind trial, neither they nor the attending physician knows. "Blindness" prevents either patient psychology or physician bias from influencing reactions and study results. For example, an investigator could subconsciously select less-sick patients for a drug that is hoped to be shown more effective than another. Generally at the start of Phase III clinical trials, there is no scientific indication that one therapy being tested is better than the other or that a third, superior treatment exists.

If, during the course of the trial, statistics based on constantly monitored data should prove that a new treatment is either highly beneficial or detrimental, the data safety and monitoring board overseeing the trial will immediately alert the investigators and the trial will be stopped. Stopping the trial at that point gives all of its participants the opportunity to avail themselves of the treatment that the statistics have shown to be the most effective.

A special category of Phase III cancer trials is known as "adjuvant trials," in which one type of cancer treatment is added to another. For example, if the standard treatment for head and neck tumor is surgery, a trial in which radiotherapy is added would be an adjuvant trial. The new therapy is usually tested in patients who have no evidence of disease after the principal treatment has been used but who are at high risk of recurrence. The added or "adjuvant" treatment represents an attempt to improve disease-free survival. The combination of two treatments must be tested in a small feasibility trial, analogous to a Phase II trial. If the combination proves safe and effective, it will be used as part of a randomized Phase III trial.

A point to remember is that the most significant breakthroughs in the history of medicine have occurred without clinically gathered statistics. A striking example is insulin therapy for diabetes. Treatments requiring huge Phase III trials usually demonstrate only that a particular therapy offers *some* improvement over another. Nevertheless, those therapies, though less dramatically verified, often do save and improve the quality of many lives.

Suzanne, one of this book's authors, could have given her mother even more help than that already described if she had known how to find and study the then ongoing clinical trials for chemotherapy regimens following colon cancer surgery. Six months after her mother's surgery (resection) for primary colon cancer, the *New England Journal of Medicine* published the results of clinical trials suggesting that a highly effective drug combination be given within weeks of resection for the particular stage of her mother's cancer.

The study's principal investigators recommended that the new drug combination be considered standard treatment to prevent metastasis. If Suzanne had read about the earlier trial phases and requested that her mother receive that particular treatment, the cancer's spread might have been stopped much sooner. Both drugs were already FDA approved and commercially available; it was the new *combination* that was tested and eventually found to be superior to previous treatments.

WHY ENTER A CLINICAL TRIAL?

Essentially, you would want to participate in a clinical trial because an innovative treatment or drug is readily available only on an investigative basis (see "Investigational Treatment without a Trial," on page 223, for other options for getting drugs awaiting FDA approval) or because you wish to contribute to the scientific knowledge of your disease.

In the first instance, you would participate in clinical research because the treatment you want is available only in the trials. You could be sure of getting that drug, however, only by taking part in a non-randomized trial. Almost always, these are Phase II trials. In Phase III trials you would stand only a fifty-fifty chance of receiving the investigative treatment. In such circumstances, it is almost impossible to predict whether your decision will prove beneficial to you. Even so, patients who have a chronic disease often participate in randomized trials in the hope that a new therapy, even if its advantages are marginal, will improve their quality of life. Doctors who help enroll them in the trials are well aware that they may have a difficult moral choice in how they advise their patients about clinical research.

"In general, I would consider experimental therapy for any patient who wanted to continue aggressive treatment and in whom current therapy had failed," says Dr. Noel Ballentine, an internist in academic medicine. "Some therapies, at least in some situations, can do more harm than good. But many patients feel that giving up and letting a disease win is worse than not trying *something*."

LOOKING FOR POSSIBLE BENEFITS

Ronald Surface, the forty-six-year-old career army officer with early-onset Parkinson's disease, as mentioned in chapter 3, found himself in this situation. Ron is a computer database and information expert who studied all the medical literature on a drug that was being tested in the treatment of Parkinson's. He felt the possible benefits were worth the risk of entering the trial, in which he might be randomized out of getting the drug or receive the drug and obtain no advantage from it.

"I was experiencing considerable discomfort," says Ron, "and was not satisfied with the effectiveness of my medications, although my physician assured me that they were the optimum treatment for a patient in my condition. After learning about

Phase III trials for a new drug and checking the information on previous clinical trials for it in the medical literature, I concluded that the drug might help me, and I volunteered for the study." Ron says the physician's assistant who served as the trial coordinator explained the consent form to him carefully. The coordinator indicated that Ron had to discontinue taking one of his medications for the duration of the trial, and also that he might receive a placebo instead of the experimental drug. Nevertheless, Ron signed the form in the hope that his condition would improve.

Unfortunately, Ron's condition worsened during his trial participation. This trial was a double-blind study, in which neither the doctor nor the patient knew whether the real drug or the placebo was being given. "Over the course of the study," Ron says, "I took steadily increasing doses of either the experimental drug or a placebo, but it apparently had little or no effect. Only the drug company knows if I was taking the new drug or a placebo."

"My condition began to deteriorate," he recalls, "and I was experiencing ever-increasing difficulty with mobility. Finally I fell and broke my ankle. Because the combination of my own medication [Ron stayed on one of his own medications, although he was asked to discontinue the other for the duration of the trial] and the trial drug did not adequately control my symptoms, I decided to withdraw from the study."

The unsuccessful outcome of Ron's experience with the study could not have been predicted. Phase III clinical trials usually run for an extended period of time. If Ron had received an effective new treatment, he would have enjoyed its advantages long before the new therapy became available to the general patient population. Moreover, even though Ron's taking part in the study did not improve his own condition, it may have indirectly benefited others through the information his case record contributes to the data. Recently, the study administrator of the trial in which he participated called Ron to tell him that the pharmaceutical company that developed the drug being tested would like to follow up patients who dropped out. "They can learn as much from the people who dropped out as they can from those who completed a trial," says Ron. "The dropouts may actually shed more light on potential side effects than the folks who had no problems."

Considering a Phase II Trial

The study that Surface entered was a Phase III trial and, as is usually the case for Phase III, it was randomized. Phase II trials are different. As already noted, they are conducted to test and measure patient response to a new therapy (not how one form of treatment compares to another). In the case of drug studies, no comparison is necessary, and *every patient in the trial is given the new drug.* If you have learned of an experimental treatment that you feel may be beneficial and it is being tested in a Phase II trial, you might consider participating.

Be aware, however, that little may be known about the new therapy at this point. The only data available in the literature will be from the Phase I trial, which studied dosages and toxicity and may have included animal studies. That information will be referenced in the Phase II protocol and found in any preliminary or pilot studies published in the pertinent journals.

Since only the treatment's safety (and some early results) will have been studied before a Phase II trial, you won't be able to make a highly informed decision about its benefits and risks. On the other hand, you will not run the chance of being randomized out of receiving the drug you want to try. Consider the alternatives carefully, and be sure to discuss them in detail with your doctor.

TRIALS FOR TREATMENTS NOT REQUIRING FDA APPROVAL

There are other clinical trials that do not require FDA approval. These include nondrug or nondevice treatments, such as the endarterectomy procedures mentioned in chapter 7. These procedures may be in trial studies to determine whether or not they should be designated as new "standard" treatments. Because they do not need FDA approval, these treatments are already available wherever physicians have been trained to provide them. Some people feel that the vigilance with which such trials are monitored will almost guarantee they themselves will get excellent care, even if they are randomized out of what is being tested as the newer "standard" therapy.

Remember, if you have decided that a specific innovative procedure offers you the best chance of recovery, you'll want to be 100 percent certain that you receive the treatment. Enrolling in a randomized trial would reduce that chance by half.

FINDING OUT ABOUT CLINICAL TRIALS

You can obtain information about ongoing clinical trials in several ways, although the process may involve networking as well as searching. If you are working with the primary care physician who diagnosed your condition and with whom you have already developed a rapport, tell him or her you would like to explore the possibility of participating in an investigative study. Your physician can help locate ongoing clinical trials in a number of ways. A doctor on staff at a medical center can ask there about trials in which they're currently participating or can place a call to such a center, even if unaffiliated with it.

If you are primarily under the care of a specialist, such as a medical oncologist, your doctor may also know of clinical trials for which you may be a candidate. If so, ask to see and study the trial information for yourself and get a second medical opinion. Resist letting any physician "steer" you toward a particular trial, especially one in which the doctor's own institution is involved. While your doctor's urging might reflect first-hand experience with a hopeful new trial, it might also reflect an institutional or personal interest. Investigators are always eager to obtain a large sample of patients for their trials, and they may be biased.

Cancer-Related Clinical Trials

For cancer protocols, either you or your physician can use a modem-equipped computer to connect with Physician's Data Query (PDQ), an information system provided by the National Cancer Institute (NCI). PDQ describes current clinical trials for any form of cancer, as well as eligibility requirements and the names of key investigators.

PDQ is readily accessible, for instance, through the Grateful Med software program. From the direct screen, follow the prompts until you get to the PDQ menu. From this point, a number of different routes lead to information on clinical trials, but each one will bring you to the right place. If you have difficulty, call the MEDLARS service desk (1-800-638-8480), and someone will walk you through. PDQ will furnish you with listings of current clinical trials containing all relevant information, including protocols, chief investigator, and so forth. Online costs for direct access to PDQ are somewhat higher than for Grateful Med. PDQ can also be reached through the Internet and CompuServe, where PDQ is a library file in the Cancer Forum. Information can be downloaded at almost no cost.

Information on trial protocols will describe the disease being treated, the name of the study and the study group, an FDA test number, supporting research, the names of the drugs or agents being tested and their chemical composition, and the name, address, and phone number of the trial's lead investigator. Use *Index Medicus* or MEDLINE to search for journal articles, using the drug name or other appropriate key word.

The National Cancer Institute's (800) 4CANCER phone number will also lead you to information from PDQ. Someone there will search for you, however, meaning that you do not control the search and are dependent upon the NCI representative. However, NCI's Cancerfax service provides the means for you to receive PDQ information on your own fax machine. Call (301) 402-5874. You can then request (by pressing a number) a list of codes for cancer types. Call back, enter the appropriate code, and you'll receive the trial information you need. There is no charge other than the telephone call.

OTHER PATHS TO TRIAL INFORMATION

There are numerous other sources of information on clinical trials.

Recall that Gary Schine secured his lead on a clinical trial through the local Leukemia Society chapter. National organizations such as the Leukemia Society of America, the Lupus Foundation, the American Parkinson's Disease Association, the American Cancer Society, and the National Arthritis Foundation all provide information on relevant clinical trials.

Local patient support groups, too, often keep track of pertinent trials and list them in newsletters or announce them at meetings. Coordinators of local clinical trials send information on trial protocols to support groups for the disease they're studying precisely because they know the materials will reach a large pool of potential subjects.

Since drug companies routinely send out press releases of trials they sponsor, newspapers are a good source of information on drugs in clinical research. The *Wall Street Journal*, for example, reports on new trials because stockholders are interested in what companies are working to develop. Very often the names of the principal investigator and the institution are included, allowing you to make direct contact and ask for more information.

Online message centers — Internet discussion groups and medical forums on commercial services — are good sources of leads. Several of the patients interviewed for this chapter remarked that locating a promising trial is often the result of networking, rather than relying on any one source.

If you are unfamiliar or uncomfortable with computers, a librarian may also be able to help you retrieve information on clinical trials through MEDLARS and also through the bulletin boards of national health-related organizations. In some libraries, the search service is free. The librarian can also help you locate Phase I and Phase II information on currently active Phase III trials.

One of the best ways to find out about clinical trials, says Ronald Surface, is to check with a medical school or teaching hospital near you and ask to be placed on their mailing list. Notices of clinical trials are often listed in their newsletters, and, especially if you have a chronic disease, you may be interested in regularly finding out about new investigative studies. Ron first heard about the trial in which he eventually participated in a newsletter from a nearby medical school.

GETTING INTO A TRIAL

If you decide you are interested in participating in a trial, your doctor can enroll you, or you can contact a principal investigator or trial coordinator yourself. This person will review your records to learn whether you qualify as a participant. The rules of scientific research dictate strict criteria. For example, you must be in the same stage of disease as other participants.

Even at this point, continue to ask questions of your contact person — the trial coordinator, investigator, or participating physician. You presumably know by now what the study is for. Find out who is sponsoring it; who reviewed and approved the protocol; who is monitoring the data for indications that the trial should be stopped. Also find out which costs of your care will be paid for by the trial's sponsor — and which by you. Patients enrolled in trials conducted by the NCI at their research center at Bethesda, Maryland, do not have to pay anything (other than transportation usually) when they are treated. And in most drug-company-sponsored trials, the drug is free. But you or your insurance company is responsible for other treatment and testing costs. You will want to know *exactly* what your costs will be.

Some large, national trials are multicenter studies, and patients can be treated through any number of institutions all over the country. In other cases, doctors in the community cooperate with regionally run trials. They can enroll patients and treat them locally. Large medical centers that are well known in particular areas of medicine are often the hub of clinical research activity, and patients receive treatment there. The NCI at Bethesda is an example. Remember that if entering a trial means staying in another city, you will have to weigh the advantages very carefully against the disadvantages. Being sick and separated from your family and friends could be an additional psychological burden.

If you become enrolled in a research study, you will generally meet with a trial coordinator, who explains the informed consent and answers all your questions. Be sure you once again review the purpose of the study, the kind of treatment you'll be getting and its probable effects, how the therapy compares to others, whether it may cause side effects or changes in your daily life, if there are any costs, what kind of therapy options you would have if you withdraw from the trial, and how long your case will be followed after the trial is over.

INVESTIGATIONAL TREATMENT WITHOUT A TRIAL

What if you have found a treatment you'd like to pursue but you do not qualify for, or choose, clinical trial enrollment? If the drug(s) are not yet cleared for marketing, discuss it with your doctor, who may agree that the treatment is a good choice and provide you with that therapy. Other options also exist.

Special Protocols

"Compassionate use" protocols are provided by the drug company or other drug sponsor in cases where a drug is nearing final approval but is not yet being marketed. "Compassionate use investigational new drug (IND) authorization" is provided to certain patients meeting specific criteria. If the FDA approves the protocol, the drug can be released on an individual basis to patients who have the disease for which the drug is being approved. Contact the drug company (not the FDA) for information on how the new protocol may be initiated, or work with your doctor to obtain the information.

In addition, for drugs related to any form of cancer but which are not yet marketed, new procedures at the FDA now enable it to provide IND authorization. In this case, the doctor must make the request directly to the FDA.

Foreign Sources

Another means of obtaining drugs not yet approved by the FDA is to arrange to import them through foreign pharmaceutical firms from countries where they are commercially available. For the last several years, the FDA has allowed doctors of patients with a serious illness to obtain such drugs on a case-by-case basis.

According to one such source in London, Alan Pharmaceuticals Ltd., a patient in the United States must obtain an imported drug directly through a physician. The doctor must make the arrangements with the foreign pharmaceutical supplier, ordering the medication with a prescription. Upon approval, the supplier will export the drugs directly to the doctor.

The *Extra Pharmacopoeia* (often known simply as "Martindale") provides an official list of medicinal drugs used throughout the world. It includes the manufacturer's name and address. If a drug not yet available in the United States is produced in other countries, it will be listed in the *Extra Pharmocopoeia*. This book, which can be found in larger medical libraries, is also an excellent source of detailed information, including journal references, on each drug listed. Also, as noted in chapter 10, the computerized database EMBASE contains much more information on European drugs than does MEDLINE.

༚

Clinical research, in the form of clinical trials, performs a service to science that can be met only by studying human responses to medical treatment in a formalized manner. There are both drawbacks and benefits to participating in them. Take careful account of all the facets of a trial. Even if you don't participate, you may learn of and obtain a treatment that might help you.

Some people decide to participate in a randomized trial not from real hope of a cure but as a contribution to medical knowledge. This can be a source of true satisfaction. As Dr. Ballentine says, "Progress from research may benefit society, even though the individual may get no benefit. Some patients do feel this is worthwhile, even if it is their last effort in life."

But clinical trials do not only offer the means to making a noble gesture at the end of life. As Ronald Surface observes, they often inspire hope:

> With thirty-eight clinical trials currently under way, as well as several surgical procedures being evaluated, there is considerable optimism that we are on the verge of a major breakthrough in the treatment, if not a cure, of Parkinson's disease. Parkinson's disease is a relentlessly progressive disorder. There would not be much to look forward to if I did not believe that continued research can make a difference.

The nature of experimental research is that some promising approaches fail, while others pay off. Clinical trials, although not appropriate for everyone, do offer a means to innovative medical therapy. Therefore, if your other choices do not seem as promising as you would wish, it's important to know how to locate information about therapies that are today experimental but tomorrow may be accepted as the newest and best standard for medical practitioners everywhere.

15.

Professional Information Searches

ELAINE, A BUSY professional in her mid-twenties, was engaged to marry a man with a serious health problem: Alport's syndrome, a form of kidney disease. Her fiancé had told her that the disease was genetically transmitted and that he might someday need a kidney transplant. She wanted to find out more: the success rates of kidney transplants, possible effects of medication, and the risk of passing on the disease to their children.

She urged her fiancé, who then lived in another city, to ask his physician more questions, and, having recently joined CompuServe, posted a notice in its Health and Fitness Forum asking how to learn more about Alport's syndrome. One of several replies came from a professional information finder who offered to research her questions for a $75 fee.

"I was working," she says, "and it was a lot easier for me to write a check than going to a library and spending hours poring through things and maybe walking away with ten percent of it being what I wanted. I thought, 'Gee, for seventy-five dollars I'd be stupid not to have him do this.' "

Elaine was pleased with the results. Within a few weeks, she received a large package (roughly seventy pages) of material, mostly photocopies of articles from medical journals. From them, she says, "We were able to figure out that if we had a son he wouldn't get it, but a daughter would have a fifty-fifty chance of having the gene." The material included "lots of stuff on transplants and drugs" and either answered her questions or provided her fiancé with points of departure for questioning his own physician. She describes the search as "targeted to my situation" and has since recommended the researcher to friends with medical questions.

COMMISSIONED SEARCHES AS AN OPTION

Hiring someone to do a search for you or to help you with a search is one option for locating medical information. You may find this approach appealing if you lack ready access to a good medical library or a personal computer, or if your time constraints or physical condition make a do-it-yourself search especially difficult. You can, by prudent planning, minimize the risk that you'll waste money. You do, however, risk missing out on the self-education that comes from exploring medical information sources on your own. Acquiring the knowledge you need for a partnership with your physician is a process, not something you can buy prepackaged.

As you might expect, the demand for specialized information has created a market niche for people who know how to find it, a class of people known as information brokers or information professionals (IPs). You can commission an IP to provide a fast overview of a medical problem or, conversely, to check for information on databases to which you lack easy access. This chapter will tell you how to locate IPs, how to assess the pros and cons of using their services, and suggest ways to get your money's worth if you decide this is a sensible choice for you.

It's important to be clear about what an IP can and cannot do. An IP can search databases for you and provide you with more or less any printed information you're prepared to pay for — bibliographic citations or full texts of presumably pertinent materials. Your ability to make good use of that information depends on how complete it is, how well it matches your needs, and your own ability to communicate with your physicians. An IP cannot diagnose, prescribe, help you interpret journal articles, or in any way replace your relationship with your doctor. In short, no one else can do your thinking for you.

DECIDING WHAT YOU WISH TO PAY FOR

"Invariably," an information professional says, "when someone first calls me, they say, 'I want to know everything there is to know about thyroid cancer.' Well, no, they don't. If someone were to go onto an expensive database, they could pay a lot of money, and probably only a small percentage of what they found would be relevant to what they really wanted to know."

Your first step, therefore, is to clarify your own needs and expectations. It makes a difference whether your goal is to enhance your ability to communicate with your doctor about a chronic, nonurgent problem or to comb the literature for every possible scrap of information about a new chemotherapy protocol. Rather than concluding, "You'll get what you pay for," it's more nearly accurate to say, "You'll probably get what you know how to ask for." Whatever approach you choose, you'll get more for your money and make a faster start toward using the information you receive if you do some background reading on your own *before* hiring a searcher rather than waiting until you receive search results.

Information brokerage services may offer anything from relatively cut-and-dried packages consisting of a few general articles and citations on a broadly defined medical problem (for example, kidney disease) to highly customized searches (for example, drugs that have proven most effective in treating Alport's syndrome in males). The standardized searches tend to be less expensive, but there's not necessarily a direct correlation between price and quality.

Several IPs specializing in medical searches offer disease-specific research packages for fees that range from around $75 to about $300. (The costs of cancer-related searches tend to be at the high end of this range because they may involve checking more —

and sometimes more expensive — databases.) For example, a 40-page search package on Parkinson's disease contained a recent review article (with 45 citations); two nontechnical articles (one published by the Food and Drug Administration, the other from a university-based medical newsletter); the results of a MEDLINE search (11 abstracts); results of a search of *Books in Print* (ten titles); names, addresses, and phone numbers of twelve patient-oriented groups dealing with Parkinson's; a few miscellaneous enclosures (excerpts from a drug manual, a medical glossary, and a *Wall Street Journal* article on the prospects of a new drug). Some groups charge much lower prices — in some cases, as little as $25 or $30 — but the samples they provided, except for an article photocopy or so, were scarcely different from materials readily available at most libraries. Some public libraries and community health centers will perform basic searches for modest fees, and these are likely to be at least as satisfactory as the simpler fixed-fee packages.

More specialized services come higher. Martha, a professional photographer in her sixties, used a progressively specific series of searches to locate information to help her communicate with physicians, who had not been able to diagnosis a problem that had often sent her to hospital emergency rooms to relieve severe choking sensations. The information retrieved by these searches helped her find a doctor who correctly diagnosed her problem as bronchiectasis, a progressive deterioration of the bronchial tubes that help air circulate throughout the lungs. Subsequent searches located articles that convinced her to accept the treatment this physician recommended, which substantially relieved her condition. Altogether, she spent five to six hundred dollars on these searches.

Could she have located the same information more cheaply herself? It would certainly seem so — assuming access to a good medical library or a modem-equipped computer. Yet like Elaine, who spent $75 for a quick report on Alport's syndrome, Martha considers her information purchases "a great bargain." She's simply delighted that she at last learned what she needed to know to secure a correct diagnosis and treatment.

One low-cost (or even no-cost, if you indicate that you cannot afford payment) source is Med Help International, a nonprofit search service, whose addresses (postal and e-mail) and phone numbers are provided in chapter 10. It is staffed by volunteers, who include physicians, other health care professionals, and active patients. Med Help International specializes in answering questions rather than providing large packages of reading material. But those answers can be time-savers: for example, a twenty-four-hour turnaround on the name of a doctor "close to Alaska" qualified in a specialized surgical procedure for trigeminal neuralgia.

LOCATING AN INFORMATION PROFESSIONAL

A few big-city Yellow Pages list IPs (usually under "Information Services"), but services so advertised are more likely to specialize in business searches than health care. You do, however, have several ways of finding a suitable searcher.

As is the case for so many information sources, one place to start is in a library, either on your own or by a phone call to a reference librarian. Magazines of the kind carried even by small-town libraries, particularly those oriented toward time-conscious business readers (like *U.S. News* and *Forbes*), often run feature articles listing and sometimes evaluating professional medical search services. Moreover, medical librarians may be able to advise you of professional searchers used by physicians in your area. (Yes, physicians do sometimes commission searches.) Unless you're looking for tutoring, however, there's little advantage to hiring a searcher from your local area. A searcher across the country has access to the same databases as one next door and can get reports to you almost as fast.

If you belong to a commercial online service, posting a notice on an appropriate bulletin board is likely to lead to contacts, either from professional searchers or, better, from individuals who are prepared to recommend searchers whose services they have used and found helpful. Don't expect a unanimous recommendation. Different participants in online forums often express quite different opinions about the same searcher.

The Association of Independent Information Professionals (AIIP), 245 Fifth Avenue, Suite 2103, New York, NY 10016, (212)

779-1855, is an organization for IPs whose members pledge to abide by a professional code of ethics. It will provide names of its members who list medical searches as a specialty.

The most comprehensive print reference on information services is the *FISCAL Directory of Fee-Based Research and Document Supply Services*, copublished by the County of Los Angeles Public Library and the American Library Association. It includes all document delivery and "library-type" research services, whether offered by libraries, trade associations, government agencies, or commercial services. The *Burwell Directory of Information Brokers* (formerly *Directory of Fee-Based Information Services*) concentrates on IPs. Both reference works are likely to be available in a good-sized public library. The Burwell directory is organized by subject specialty, but only a few of its approximately one thousand listed searchers identify themselves as specializing in medical information.

SELECTING AN INFORMATION PROFESSIONAL

Locating names of qualified searchers isn't likely to be a major problem. The more important questions are how to pick the right person for you and how to make the most effective use of his or her services.

Because information brokerage is a relatively new field, there are no licensing requirements for practitioners. If you decide to use an IP, you'll have to use your own best judgment on selecting a particular individual or service, just as you should in choosing a physician. You should do the following:

• Find out how long the service has been in business. New services may be reliable, but a track record is one indicator of customer satisfaction and probably of quality.

• Find out the IP's training or experience, particularly in medical specialties. Someone trained as a reference librarian with background in a medical field would theoretically be ideal. Completion of one of the National Library of Medicine seminars on searching MEDLARS databases is a modest plus, but note that these are only one-week sessions.

• Ask if the service will guarantee its results and what that guarantee means. Some services contacted indicate that they will refund a dissatisfied client's money (after getting their report back), with no questions asked. Others will do second searches without charge when some basic search assumption has changed for reasons the client could not reasonably have foreseen, such as a physician's changing an initial diagnosis.

• Make sure your contract with an IP contains a satisfactory confidentiality agreement. Most IPs say they keep client names confidential as a matter of course, but you should be clear on this.

• Have a firm understanding in advance about what you'll get and what you'll pay for it. How many full-text articles can you expect to get, as distinct from citations or abstracts you'll need to look up for yourself? What will be the mix of articles from general publications and from medical journals? Most important, what do *you* want? The authority of professional journal articles? The ease of reading material from popular sources? Or some mix of both?

• Pay attention to the questions the IP asks *you*. He or she should help you to focus your inquiry. Otherwise, you could end up with a long printout of citations that bear little relationship to the specific information you need.

• Establish how soon you will get your search results. This may be negotiable, depending on your needs and the searcher's other commitments.

• Ask if follow-up searches are done at reduced rates, in case you want to pursue some topic in depth or want a later update on some issue.

• Ascertain whether search reports are confined to mainstream medicine or whether they include articles on "alternative" therapies. It's up to you whether you want information on diet and nutrition, folk remedies, acupuncture, or other topics outside the usual scope of clinical literature.

THE PROS AND CONS OF COMMISSIONED SEARCHES

Information professionals, not surprisingly, say that their searches are likely to be more comprehensive and more efficient than those done by amateurs.

IPs subscribe to a number of computerized databases. Although you have relatively easy access to the largest and most valuable medical database, MEDLINE, access to others can be expensive. If, for example, you were interested in a report on interactions between two relatively new drugs, it makes sense to consult EMBASE. You can do that yourself via IQUEST on CompuServe, but you could easily run up a search bill well in excess of what you'd pay a pro. "Every database has its own unique way of searching," says one professional, "and unless you are familiar with that database and search it continuously, it's very likely you'll not be able to do the best search you can do. If you're depending on it for your health and your life, I'd recommend having someone doing it who uses it on a daily basis."

In practice, however, searchers do most of their searching on MEDLINE and in readily available print references mentioned elsewhere in this book. One San Francisco organization, Planetree, maintains file folders of materials on diseases and procedures, primarily for community people who walk in to do their own searches. But Planetree staff will also do searches on request, charging very modest fees for copies of materials the group already has on hand and, for customized MEDLINE searches, fees comparable to those of commercial services.

A conscientious and skilled IP can help you define your questions. At least one searcher says that she always tries to talk to a potential client by telephone even when a written request seems clear; the conversation helps her feel more confident that she understands the person's needs.

The downside of hiring someone for a search is that you risk missing important aspects of your own education. Finding the best treatment is likely to be almost inseparable from your own involvement in the search process. You're not just searching libraries and databases but exploring a world in which a lot of information is provided by people with whom you come in contact. Much of the value of online searching, for example, is that it exposes you to many points of view and gives you practice in formulating and refining questions. You no more want to be totally dependent on one IP for your window on this world than on one M.D.

This book's authors feel that you should *not* hire an IP out of simple insecurity about your own information-finding skills. If you feel you need coaching in computers or help with medical reference sources, consider tutoring. A university library science department may be able to recommend promising graduate students, or a medical librarian at a teaching hospital may be able to identify a second-year or third-year medical student with good search skills.

Whether or when it makes sense for you to use an IP depends entirely on your own circumstances. If you're physically unable to do much searching for yourself or are unable to spare the time to do so, consider hiring someone rather than doing without information you need for a dialogue with your physician. You should also consider hiring a professional if, on the basis of some preliminary searching on your own, you have reason to believe that a crucial piece of information may be especially hard to find.

Whether doing your own searching, commissioning searches, or some combination of the two, think of *information-assimilation* as a process, not of *information* as a product that you can simply find or buy and then be done with it. As one experienced searcher says: "You can't drink by the bucketful. Go to the well early and often."

16.

Coping with HMOs and Other Insurers

IN THE WORDS of a recent *Wall Street Journal* article, "Unlimited choice of doctors is steadily going the way of house calls." All insurers have always imposed limits on what treatments they will pay for, but managed care insurers (commonly known as HMOs, for "health maintenance organizations") also impose limits on your access to providers.

This can be bad news for you as an active patient because it may limit your ability to receive the treatment you believe is best for you. In some instances, innovative treatment options are performed at only a few places; in other instances, even if the treatment you think best is available through a facility covered by your insurance plan, you may want to pursue it only if it can be provided by a physician or surgeon whose track record you know to be outstanding. Recall the case of Bob Long in chapter 7, in which an endarterectomy was a prudent choice only if performed by a surgical team with a low record of complications.

This chapter offers you an overview of how the two major kinds of insurance plans work. It describes the opposite economic biases built into each of them and explains how these biases may (not necessarily, but *may*) affect the quality of medical services that you receive. Finally, and most important, it suggests ways for you to maximize your chances of getting the treatment of your choice from the physician of your choice.

When you're seriously ill, insurance and paperwork are the last things you want to worry about, but, unfortunately, they can be a major factor in medical decisions. Keep in mind that the legal and economic contexts within which you pursue your search for the best treatment can change at any time. As noted at the beginning of this book, rapid change is a fact of life in all aspects of medicine. Changes in scientific knowledge and treatment technologies usually work to your benefit. That's not necessarily true for changes in the politics and economics of health care delivery, but your willingness to take charge of crucial decisions can tilt the odds in your favor.

Under any conceivable health care delivery or health care finance system, however, one rule is sure to hold good: *the more you understand, both about treatment options and the systems within which people who provide treatments work, the better off you are.*

EXAMPLES OF HOW KNOWLEDGE CAN PAY OFF

Consider, for example, the story of Estelle Zevola, a Pennsylvania woman who suffered from a rare disease that attacks the liver, amyloidosis. In May 1993, Zevola's insurer, an HMO, told her that it would not pay for a liver transplant because the procedure was "experimental" for amyloidosis.

Refusing to accept this "no" as final, Zevola's sister-in-law, Joyce Zevola, "spent hours in medical libraries researching the rare disease and on the phone with amyloidosis researchers," according to an Associated Press news story. Joyce located a journal article supporting Zevola's claim that a liver transplant appeared to be the best treatment available. The article had not even been published when the HMO first considered the case. It had appeared in the May issue of a British medical journal, *The Lancet,* a scant two weeks before Joyce found it. Moreover, Pennsylvania Governor Robert Casey had received a successful liver transplant for the same condition. (The governor also received a heart transplant.) Confronted with this evidence and under pressure from the media, the insurer reversed its position. Maybe Zevola would have won her case without publicity, maybe not. But *not even Governor Casey* would have received the best available treatment if *his* doctors had not been current on the pertinent medical literature.

Consider also a footnote to the story of Al Musella, the podiatrist whose database searches on behalf of Janet, a family member suffering from a potentially fatal brain tumor, led him to a journal article indicating that a drug normally used to combat breast cancer also showed great promise for certain brain tumors. The drug was not only expensive; the remarkable success rate reported in the medical journal was based on administering the drug at approximately ten times its normal dosage. Janet's insurer, also an HMO, although one with fairly flexible rules on patient choice, declined to pay for a treatment it considered experimental.

The treatment *was* experimental, and Musella did not try to argue that point. He did persuade the insurer to pay for the standard dosage used for breast cancer therapy (that is, approximately 10 percent of the total cost). Using his knowledge of drug company policies, he also persuaded the manufacturer to donate another 10 percent to Janet and still another 10 percent to her doctor as a professional sample. Altogether, Janet would be reimbursed for about 30 percent of the drug's cost. (Musella says that the drug company would have been more generous but feared to appear to be promoting an untested application of its product.)

A few months later, Musella was able to report to Janet's insurer that Janet was responding to the innovative treatment with what seemed an almost miraculous recovery. The insurer immediately reversed its initial refusal and did so without quibbles. "As long as it's working, we'll pay," an HMO official told Musella.

For the patients involved in these two insurance controversies, the key to success was their medical knowledge and their ability to make a case based on that knowledge. One case was decided in the glare of media publicity, the other quietly and without controversy. The common element was homework done by the patients and their advocates, who had thoroughly researched the *medical* issues involved and were able to show that the very latest medical findings lent support to their positions.

TWO TYPES OF INSURANCE COVERAGE

Health insurance plans tend to fall into two major categories: third-party payer plans and managed care plans. Hundreds of variations exist within each category, as do various kinds of hybrids. But understanding the main features of each plan will be enough to help you to make rational choices when you can and to be alert for problems when your choices are limited.

Third-party payer plans include that class of policies that many people still think of simply as "insurance" — that is, the kind of insurance held, until a few years ago, by almost everyone with any health insurance at all. This form of insurance is called "third-party" insurance because the insurer is the third of three distinct parties involved: (1) the patient, (2) the health care providers (physicians and hospitals), and (3) the insurer. As a patient you pay a periodic premium that covers the costs of treatment from any provider of your choice, subject to deductibles and many other limits that vary from policy to policy. Doctors and hospital administrators usually refer to third-party payer insurance as a "fee-for-service" plan because that term describes how they get paid: according to a fee schedule for specified types and levels of service — for example, so much money per office visit, per X-ray, per appendectomy, and so on.

"Managed care" refers to a type of insurance in which you, or whoever has selected your insurance, trade off some of your freedom to choose physicians in exchange for other benefits, primarily lower costs. The most familiar term for this kind of insurer is "HMO," although, strictly speaking, an HMO is only one kind of managed care plan. (This chapter will use the terms "HMO" and "managed care" interchangeably.)

Under a managed care plan, a single legal entity assumes responsibility both for paying for health care and, directly or indirectly, for providing it. The roles of provider and insurer are to some extent combined: the insurer assumes some of the responsibility for the quality of care delivered, and the physician assumes some of the financial risk involved in covering its costs. As an HMO member, you pay the HMO a periodic fee, just as you would to a third-party insurance company, plus a small fee per office visit. But the HMO will pay only for services provided by physicians on its approved list.

In a managed care plan, the first physician you see is known as a "primary care provider" (PCP). This physician is paid according to the number of HMO members he or she agrees to accept as potential patients rather than according to the quantity of services the physician actually provides. Insurers and doctors call this form of reimbursement a "capitation" (per head) plan, as distinct from a fee-for-service plan. (In a few HMOs, called "staff-model" HMOs, physicians are employees of the HMO and hence on salary.)

For medical specialists, however, most managed care plans pay on a fee-for-service basis. The plans manage the cost of specialist services by using the PCPs as "gatekeepers." That is, your PCP, who may be either a single physician or a group practice, provides your mandatory point of entry to the HMO system. Unless he or she refers you to a specialist, you will not be reimbursed for seeing one. Normally, you will receive full reimbursement only for the services of specialists on the HMO's approved list.

Managed care plans have expanded dramatically in recent years, at the expense of third-party payer plans. During the last decade, HMO enrollment quadrupled. By the end of 1994, approximately 50 percent of all Americans with prepaid health care coverage were receiving this coverage under some form of managed care. Most of this expansion in managed care has resulted from the growth of for-profit entities, primarily those associated with insurance companies.

The reason for the expansion of managed care plans is that they cost less than third-party payer policies. An HMO can use its buying power as the economic representative of thousands of patients to negotiate favorable prices (and, ideally, a uniformly high standard of service) from physicians, hospitals, and pharmacies. It passes part of those savings on to its members. But its bargaining power depends on its ability to refuse to pay providers who aren't on its approved list. This, of course, in turn means that patients who want to go to off-list providers must pay all or part of the costs of doing so — the percentage depending on the terms of the particular HMO contract. In an economic sense, joining an HMO is much like joining a union: union members gain collective bargaining power but lose individual discretion in negotiating their own employment terms.

HOW INSURANCE PLANS MAY AFFECT YOUR CARE

If you get your insurance through a small employer, you may have little practical choice between a third-party plan and a managed care plan. Even so, what you don't know about your insurance could be as hazardous to your health as any other gap in your knowledge.

If you do have a choice among insurance plans, you'd like to retain as much flexibility as possible. How you choose plans will depend on factors only you can know: your age, your finances, and your assessment of your health risks. If you could somehow know that you'd never become sick or injured, you would carry no insurance at all. If you could know that you'd enjoy general good health or contract only illnesses without complications, you would choose an HMO. If you could know that you'd soon be diagnosed with an illness requiring long and costly treatment, you would pay whatever is necessary to buy a plan with virtually unlimited coverage. That none of us can know what the future holds is what makes some form of insurance prudent and makes the choice among policies difficult. In the face of uncertainty, you'd surely like to preserve your ability to consult those physicians and select those treatments you believed to be best for you, assuming that you could afford such a plan.

Here's a quick summary of how insurance plans relate to the personal and economic interests of the three parties already mentioned — patients, insurers, and providers.

You, as a *patient*, naturally want the best treatment at the lowest possible cost. "Best" means neither too little nor too much. You neither want to be denied care that you need nor to be subjected to unnecessary medication, unnecessary X-rays, or unnecessary surgery.

An *insurer's* role under any plan is by definition a purely economic role, for any insurer's goal is to make a profit or, in the case of a not-for-profit entity, to at least break even after expenses. Again, your concerns as a patient are both price and quality of service. Sooner or later, all insurers have market incentives to satisfy customers on both of these points, but at any given time *any* insurer may serve its customers badly on either or both of them. An HMO may be a not-for-profit entity, as many are, but that provides no guarantee that its managers will make good use of their resources. Not-for-profits are subject to the same marketplace pressures as for-profit organizations, largely because they can attract first-class physicians only by paying market rates.

For *providers* (doctors, pharmacists, and hospitals) the economic incentives associated with the two different kinds of plans are as different as day and night. Under fee-for-service plans, doctors as a class have an economic interest in providing as many billable services as possible (consultations, drugs, tests, or surgery), and individual doctors may have specific conflicts of interest (for example, ownership of test facilities, close personal relationships with specialists, or dependence on other doctors for referrals to their own practice). Considering only economics and ignoring most doctors' strong personal and professional ethics, the principal restraints on overtreating patients are fear of malpractice suits and insurers' unwillingness to pay for excessive levels of "care."

Under managed care plans, primary care physicians share an insurer's interests in keeping the total level of patient services down. As a class, HMO primary care physicians risk conflicts of interest: the necessity of working within a cost-control structure that tempts them to provide less care than a patient may need. Some plans create direct conflicts by forcing primary care doctors to pay for certain diagnostic services out of their own pockets. Others contain more general incentives to economize — for example, bonuses to doctors whose annual per-patient costs for certain services are significantly below the HMO average. Either way, for doctors paid on a capitation basis, an ideal economic world would be similar to an insurer's ideal — that is, one in which many are enrolled but few need treatment.

Managed care, therefore, makes it harder for you to find a physician-ally who will fight with you for what you are convinced is the best treatment, especially if that treatment is expensive or unconventional. From the perspective of whoever pays your insurance premiums, that's an advantage: primary care physicians are unable to consider treatment costs as an insurer's problem and hence are less likely to consistently interpret gray areas in insurers' rules in their patients' favor. For patients, who understandably feel that they need every possible break and hence need insurers' gray areas interpreted in their favor, that's a potential problem.

HOW HMOS HANDLE PATIENTS

In almost all cases, the HMO gatekeeper of record will be a general practitioner, an internist, a family physician, a pediatrician, or sometimes a specialist in obstetrics and gynecology. Normally, HMOs permit you to choose this doctor from anyone on their approved list and, if you aren't satisfied, to switch to another doctor on their list, usually on request.

The busier doctors become, the more likely they are to delegate aspects of screening patients to nurses or other non-M.D.s. It has been suggested that managed care plans lead to more such delegation because doctors who are reimbursed according to the number of patients they accept tend to accept more than they can readily handle. This may be so, but decisions of this kind depend on how your doctor chooses to operate — *not* the kind of insurance you happen to have. If you are asked questions by a nurse that you would expect to be asked by a physician, the most appropriate response is (a) to answer the questions with as much thoroughness as possible and (b) to make sure that you repeat those answers to the physician. Try to think of it as two chances to get your symptoms and prior medical history on the record.

If your PCP agrees that you need to consult a specialist, you'll be given names of approved specialists within your geographical area. If you want someone else, the burden of proving your need to "go out of plan" will fall on you. You'll almost certainly need the support of your PCP to succeed. You'll probably have to argue the case in terms of the out-of-plan specialist's special expertise rather than implying that the in-plan specialists are generally less competent.

DEMONSTRATING MEDICAL NECESSITY

Any insurer — conventional or HMO — will insist on some documentation that a treatment is medically necessary. "Medically necessary" means that *you* need a treatment because it has been shown to be useful in treating conditions like yours and seems most appropriate for *your* condition, compared to other available alternatives. This is not the same as a "covered treatment," which refers only to any of a class of treatments for which an insurer has agreed to pay when the treatment is shown to be necessary. For example, your policy may cover massage therapy, but your physician must still document that you need it.

Insurers contend that physicians' failure to document medical necessity is often the reason for denial of treatment. Doctors, confident of their own diagnoses and prescriptions, may simply assert claims that an insurer feels they should justify. For example, an HMO claims examiner who specializes in reviewing appeals of denied mental health care benefits, says flatly that

> patients aren't getting their full benefits because the provider didn't provide enough information, or the right kind of information, or accurate information. It's not enough to say someone has "dysthymia," or an "underlying depression."

The examiner further notes that the psychologist should provide a description of how that patient fits into such a diagnosis; also how the illness affects his life adversely. The examiner continues:

> A person may have a twenty-year depression and have low self-esteem, but if they're the president of a company, appropriately parenting, and functional in many ways, it may be a luxury to continue counseling. That is, it may not be considered medically necessary even if there are the symptoms to back it up.

She adds: "Some of our psychologists and psychiatrists enjoy working with an HMO. They do a good job on the forms. They communicate with us by phone. Others don't, and their patients don't get as much service."

Requiring that your physician document medical necessity is generally in your best interest; for example, it makes it harder for a careless or unscrupulous doctor to profit from removing your healthy appendix or uterus. Physicians, however, complain that insurers' rules for documenting medical necessity may be unclear or inconsistent. No doubt both the insurers and the doctors have a point. But the problem for you remains the same if you are denied a treatment option. Whether the problem results from an insurer's being vague about its decision rules or a doctor's being less than diligent in documenting your need, in the end, you may have to help provide the documentation yourself.

Unfortunately, the physician who has the qualifications you need as a medical specialist may regard insurance-related paperwork as an unpleasant necessity to be dealt with as summarily as possible. You may still want that physician to treat you — indeed, you *should* prefer a physician whose professional life is built around, say, finding the best chemotherapy to one whose orientation is filling out forms. But you should also find a behind-the-scenes way to make sure that paperwork on your behalf is always adequately prepared.

This is another area where research in primary medical literature may pay off. If you have to appeal a denial of treatment, your goal will be to show that the treatment you seek is *medically necessary*. And you may well win. An attorney commissioned by a state medical society to analyze physician disputes with the insurance giant Blue Shield concluded that the insurer's review committees, composed of physicians, were generally open-minded to arguments presented on medical grounds. ("They can make mistakes," he wrote, "but there does not appear to be an intentional disregard of the presentation made by the provider if it is a clinical presentation.")

SEEKING LEGAL HELP

If you must challenge a policy as unfair, or if you believe your medical arguments are being unreasonably rejected, you need legal help. All insurers are sensitive both to the direct costs of large jury awards and to the resulting political damage stemming from bad publicity. HMOs are particularly sensitive because their negligence and mistakes draw pointed attacks from organized physician groups as well as patient advocacy organizations. You've doubtless read horror stories about lifesaving treatments denied by HMOs and other insurers, most of which become a matter of record only after litigation.

For example, in 1991 Nelene Fox developed a breast cancer that spread to her bone marrow. Some of the physicians she consulted said she was an appropriate candidate for a bone marrow transplant. Her HMO insurer, Health Net, a division of HN Management Holdings, contended that the benefits of the procedure were unproved. Nelene died. In December, 1993, a jury in Riverside, California, found that Health Net had been guilty of bad faith, breach of contract, and recklessly inflicted emotional distress. The jury ordered Health Net to pay to the Fox estate damages totaling $89.3 million. (This total included $77 million in punitive damages; the purpose of punitive damages is to deter future wrongdoing, as distinct from compensating victims for actual suffering.) This award was the largest ever against an insurer for refusal to provide health coverage benefits. (After Health Net announced its intention to appeal, the parties agreed in April 1994 to a settlement, reducing the jury award by an undisclosed amount.)

Although judgments of this size are rare, attorneys specializing in these areas say that settlements are common. One such attorney was quoted in a 1994 *Wall Street Journal* article as saying that he had won all of his 250 cases, only eight of which went to trial.

One element of advocacy is the skilled use of publicity. Estelle Zevola, who won payment for a liver transplant, was almost certainly helped by media publicity of the fact that within a month of her denial, Pennsylvania Governor Robert P. Casey had received a heart-liver transplant. But she also had the latest research at her fingertips.

"TRUST, BUT VERIFY": A SEVEN-POINT SUMMARY

An adversarial approach should always be a last resort. No matter how you analyze the economics of health care and the rules of your particular insurer, one point merits reemphasis: *Under any doctor-patient-insurer arrangement whatsoever, your first priority should be to establish good human relationships with the people involved.*

If you have a conventional health insurance policy, don't walk into your doctor's office expecting him or her to run up the biggest bill possible. If you're in an HMO, don't walk in expecting to be denied care that you need. Start from the assumption that you and your physician are committed to a common goal — providing you with the best possible treatment within whatever financial rules your insurance coverage may impose. And attempt to deal with insurers on the premise that they want to honor their commitments and do their part to help you get well quickly, both because they are staffed by decent people and because, as business entities, they have reputations to consider.

Nevertheless, things can go wrong when you're dealing with organizations, even those staffed by conscientious, well-intentioned people. Keep in mind the proverb former president Ronald Reagan used to describe his approach to disarmament negotiations with the former Soviet Union: "Trust, but verify."

To that end, here are seven suggestions:

1. Make every effort to get your physicians on your side, starting with your primary care provider. Show that you're prepared to be an active patient and respect the pressures on that physician, especially the pressures of time and paperwork. In short, establish a working relationship based on mutual respect. You're going to need the PCP not only for routine care but, potentially, as an advocate for specialist services.

2. If you decide that that kind of relationship isn't going to be possible with your primary care physician, choose another one soon, before any adverse recommendations become a matter of record. Your HMO will almost always let you change a primary care physician; if it doesn't, you may have to pay out of your own pocket for a medical mentor.

3. Make sure you know the insurer's rules on coverage, as well as appeals procedures. For this kind of information, contact your insurer's administrative offices rather than taking up your doctor's time or defining your relationship with him in terms of insurance matters. If the material you get from your insurer doesn't answer your questions, check with the appropriate state regulatory agency. In almost all states, insurers are regulated by

two kinds of state departments. Typically, regulators in health departments deal with quality-of-care issues; those in insurance departments deal with financial and consumer issues.

4. Even when your PCP agrees that you need exceptional treatment, you may need to provide unobtrusive help in making the case for it. This could include providing your doctor with *your* written statement of symptoms, copies of journal articles, or other materials he or she may not have had time to locate. *You should no more assume that your physician will be an effective advocate than that your attorney would be an effective clinical diagnostician.*

The HMO appeals reviewer quoted earlier emphasizes that patients can help a PCP make their case by providing their own narrative or backup documentation. In the case of a child, she says, "maybe a schoolteacher will write a letter. If it all comes in together, those are the denials we'll overturn."

5. If you become involved in advocacy on your own or a family member's behalf, learn the key concepts and terms needed to make your case effectively. For example, a "covered treatment" must still be shown to be "medically necessary." You would look foolish arguing that you are entitled to a treatment simply because it is "covered."

6. Keep clinical, economic, and legal arguments separate in your own mind, and see that each argument is addressed to the appropriate audience at the appropriate stage in the decision process. You won't convince an insurer's medical review board that a nonstandard treatment is medically necessary by arguing that the insurer's paperwork procedures are unreasonable. But an insurance executive, sensitive to public relations, might accept an argument about procedural fairness when he would never second-guess a physician panel's medical judgment.

7. Never idly threaten litigation or adverse publicity, but get competent legal advice as soon as it's clear you may need it. How soon is that? You have to decide, taking into account the urgency of your medical situation and how confident you feel in your and your doctor's abilities to cooperate toward an acceptable outcome. Whatever you do, keep good records.

YOUR MEDICAL KNOWLEDGE BECOMES EVEN
MORE IMPORTANT

As this book is written, the entire health care industry is in a state of flux. Whatever happens in political arenas or the marketplace, it's unlikely that doctors will become less busy or that pressures for cost controls will be relaxed. Amid the sound and fury, remember the main point: whatever kind of insurance you have now or in the future, your own knowledge of your *medical* options will be more important than ever.

It may seem odd to suggest that you should put increased effort into exploring medical choices when your scope for acting on what you learn may be narrowing. The truth is that you'll need to know *more* about your medical options precisely because you won't be able to count on the semiautomatic support of your primary care physician for specialist referrals. And if the first specialist you consult isn't helpful, you may have to pay for consultations with other physicians yourself.

Consumers — meaning, of course, patients — have always had an uphill battle in the medical marketplace. There are many reasons for this, but one of the most important is that their understanding of the *medical* issues crucial to their treatments has been limited. It hardly mattered how knowledgeable or savvy patients might be in other areas of their lives if, faced with serious illness, they had to resign themselves to being told, by a physician, "This is what you have to do" or, by an insurer, "Your policy won't pay for that."

Your decision to become an active, informed patient will help to change that pattern for you and your family. Even if you have to make compromises on the basis of either economics or medical uncertainty, you'll be able to make those compromises intelligently, with a real sense of what you're giving up and what you're gaining. Finally, although this isn't your main goal, you and people like you may even help to improve the health care system. Physicians can be expected to become increasingly responsive to active, questioning patients. And insurers, in order to attract and keep the business of intelligent, informed consumers, will increasingly have to compete on both price and quality of medical service.

17.

Choosing Hospitals and Physicians

THE OPENING CHAPTER of this book emphasizes how fast medical knowledge changes. By now, you have doubtless realized that *access to medical knowledge* is also changing — almost always in your favor. It's a revolution that has profound implications for your search for the best treatment.

A physician and research fellow at the Harvard Medical School's Center for Clinical Computing sums up his perspective on the near future of medicine to a *Wall Street Journal* reporter like this: "The bottom line is, the consumers will have virtually all the information the professionals have."

Of course, a patient's information cannot be effective unless combined with a physician's professional training and experience. But having information makes it easier for you to become an active partner with your doctor. Information-finding skills will serve you well over time, although the state of medical knowledge itself will continue to change. It also seems likely that true doctor-patient partnerships may become far more common than they have been in the past. "The single thing you can count on [from your own medical searches] is a better relationship with a good physician," says a former reference librarian who has assisted in many searches. "When doctors see that you know what you're talking about, they feel comfortable talking to you and uncomfortable not talking to you." The Harvard physician adds, "The whole structure of medicine has been based on the assumption that physicians have the current information and patients don't. . . . Once people start getting good communication, you won't be able to play the game in the same way."

There are signs that this is beginning to happen. Previously inaccessible infomedicine resources are beginning to become more accessible and found in more useful formats. This chapter addresses two crucial and related issues — choosing a hospital and choosing a physician-specialist — noting where statistical information exists to supplement (but never replace) advice from informed professionals.

CHOOSING A HOSPITAL

Hospitals are complex institutions that bring together an extraordinary array of high technology and human skills. They cannot be evaluated as decisively as a new drug or surgical technique. Moreover, hospitals may change over time for better or for worse.

Your best source of information on hospitals is usually your own physician. His or her opinion, after all, is likely to be based on frequent firsthand observations sharpened by professional training. Moreover, your physician knows what other doctors say about hospitals to which they refer patients and can apply their comments to your situation. In some instances, however, a physician may have personal or financial reasons for preferring one facility over another or may not have had occasion to learn much about local hospitals other than those with which he or she has affiliation. If you feel that your doctor is recommending a particular facility without careful consideration of how well it meets your needs, you should not hesitate to ask for an explanation of why he feels as he does before seeking a second opinion. Remind your doctor that you want to be informed and involved in all major treatment decisions. You should discuss the choice of facilities with both your primary care physician and any specialists involved.

Your choice among treatment facilities may be dictated either by the preferences of the physician you wish to perform a procedure or by the nature of the procedure itself. For example, if you require surgery that relies on the skills of one outstanding surgeon, the individual will play the larger role, and you will probably want to go to the hospital this doctor suggests. There may be good reason to prefer one hospital over another, such as the quality of a surgical team, and you should follow your doctor's cue. If your physician has appointments at several hospitals and expresses no preference, choose on the basis of your own convenience and sense of well-being.

If the most important element is the procedure itself — for example, a bone marrow transplant, which requires a large team — you will want the institution where the best teams have compiled the best records. In that case, you can call the hospital, or ask the doctor, for the number of such procedures the facility performs monthly or annually, mortality statistics, and follow-up figures. You're entitled to this information; an institution that's proud of its record won't hesitate to make it available. In this era, when hospitals are competing for patients, you should take your time to research the record of an institution. Try to talk to people who have been there, and with physicians and medical teams who serve there.

In some instances, you may require a procedure that only one, or a few, doctors practice. Suzanne, a coauthor of this book, was able to help her mother by finding the surgeon who had himself developed a special technique for operating on liver tumors, as described in chapter 7. This doctor was the unique specialist required, and Suzanne had no problem in making the necessary arrangements. As noted earlier, however, being reimbursed for the services of a particular specialist can be difficult under managed health care, and your success will depend on how convincingly you can make your case that the special techniques of the individual you select are such as to make this physician's use "medically necessary." Your best asset will be an in-depth study of medical literature, for even the most cost-conscious insurers will not readily risk liability for major mistakes if the record shows that a patient made a strong case for a probably superior, even if nonstandard, treatment option.

STATISTICAL INFORMATION ON HOSPITALS

Most hospitals are regularly evaluated, and the results of those evaluations are increasingly becoming available to the public. What follows are two possible sources of statistical information — less rich and detailed than a physician's recommendations, but valuable nevertheless.

First, the Joint Commission on Accreditation of Health Care Organizations evaluates and accredits more than eleven thousand health care organizations in the United States, including more than 5,200 hospitals. This is roughly 80 percent of the hospitals in the country, and these hospitals account for 96 percent of patient admissions. The commission's evaluations are based on more than seven hundred standards relating to quality of care. These include patient care functions, quality of medical and other staff, and environmental safety issues, such as infection control.

Summaries of the Joint Commission's reports have been available to the public only since 1994. They show a hospital's numerical scores on about thirty measures of quality. They also show how many evaluated institutions scored within specified ranges. Each summary is accompanied by explanations of how the scores are derived.

The commission's reports now cost $30 for each hospital and may be ordered from the commission at One Renaissance Boulevard, Oakbrook Terrace, Illinois 60181, (708) 916-5800. You may be able to get them directly from hospitals in which you are interested.

A second potential source of information is reports by state agencies, some of which will be more detailed than commission reports. Thirty-five states have agencies that collect data on hospitals. For example, the Pennsylvania Health Care Cost Containment Council, less than ten years old, issues periodic reports on the frequency and *outcomes* of treatments, shown on a hospital-by-hospital basis. The treatments are listed by diagnosis-related groups (DRGs) — for example, "cardiac valve procedure with pump and without cardiac catheterization." (About 500 DRGs are used by federal and state agencies in classifying Medicare and Medicaid claims. The Pennsylvania reports cover about sixty DRGs, chosen because they are either those most often performed or, alternatively, the most expensive.)

These reports show the number of times a procedure has been performed during a year. This is important because "high-volume" hospitals that have greater experience and practice in a procedure generally have better track records. Two recent Duke University studies on angioplasty, an invasive treatment used to open up plaque-clogged arteries, reported in the *New England Journal of Medicine* and in the *Annals of Internal Medicine*, strongly suggest that deaths from complications following angioplasty occur less frequently at hospitals that have a high volume of these procedures, compared to low-volume hospitals.

The Pennsylvania reports also cover outcome data (again, by DRG): average patient stay, deaths, and a somewhat complex morbidity factor that basically reflects how well patients fared a week after the treatment in question was performed. The reports show both the hospital's actual numerical rating and a comparison with an *expected* rating based on the performance of other hospitals in its area. Notes explain how data are statistically adjusted. To take an obvious example, hospitals that admit an exceptionally high number of elderly patients can be expected to have a higher number of deaths from almost any serious procedure, and the council's "expected" death rates are adjusted to take age into account. (The council also issues treatment-oriented reports, such as *A Consumer Guide to Coronary Artery Bypass Graft Surgery*, comparing the track records of hospitals in that procedure.)

Not all states provide such detailed reports on hospitals, but the national trend is in the direction of more openness and public access. You may be able to get similar information from an agency in your state. Your starting point should be your state department of health.

EVALUATING PHYSICIANS

In choosing specialist physicians, you should try to ask other doctors or nurses to name the two or three specialists whom they would pick for themselves if they had your medical problem or were planning to undergo a procedure for which you are scheduled. Inquiring outright whether a doctor is "good" is not the best approach, since physicians will generally avoid calling a fellow doctor a *poor* choice. They will usually emphasize those who are *good* choices in a way that will be quite clear to you. This approach was the one used by the authors of *The Best Doctors in America* in preparing their list of over seven thousand top physicians nationwide in more than 350 specialties. If you have the option, consider selecting a doctor on the faculty of an academic medical center. Such physicians devote much of their professional careers to teaching and research. Publication records may provide additional clues to a physician's standing in his or her field.

It is, of course, impossible to evaluate individual professionals by statistical methods, even if there were a consensus on criteria and reporting standards. As chapter 5 explains, you can check the *ABMS Directory of Board Certified Medical Specialists* to determine if a specialist is listed there, which provides evidence of peer-evaluated advanced training. But no database purports to rank individual physicians' skills, nor should you trust one if someone were to decide to publish it.

On the negative side of physician performance, you may want to know about past problems, especially of a serious nature. Statistical information of that kind is now collected in a national database, but it is not open to public access.

With the passage of the Health Care Quality Improvement Act of 1986 (Public Law 99-660), the U.S. Congress created a National Practitioners Data Bank (NPDB), which you may have heard referred to as the "National Malpractice Data Bank," an incorrect label, but one that does partially describe its contents. The NPDB, which began operations in 1990, is maintained by a branch of the U.S. Public Health Service. Under the law, the following four classes of actions must be reported to the NPDB:

• adverse clinical privilege actions of more than 30 days taken by a hospital, HMO, or other health care organization against a doctor or dentist;

• revocation, restriction, or suspension of a doctor's or dentist's license by a state medical or dental board;
• adverse membership actions taken by professional societies against physicians or dentists;
• medical malpractice payments, currently of any amount, made on behalf of a physician, dentist, or other licensed health care practitioner to settle a judgment or claim.

By 1995, the NPDB contained the names of about 11,500 health care practitioners who had been subject to some adverse action in almost 18,000 separate cases (most often a license suspension by peer review committees, state boards, or specialty boards). It also contained the names of 64,000 professionals, mostly physicians, who lost or settled malpractice claims.

Physicians listed in the NPDB are allowed to attach a brief statement (about 75 words) of their side of the story to any entry in their files. About 12 percent of the adverse actions are disputed, as are about 6 percent of the malpractice listings. Note that physicians and their organizations have often objected to inclusion of malpractice settlements, pointing out that they and their insurers may choose to settle "nuisance" suits that they believe are without merit to avoid the time, expense, and publicity of litigation.

Hospitals *must* query the data bank when they consider a physician or other health care professional for a medical staff appointment or credentials. They must check on existing staff at two-year intervals. Certain other organizations *may* query the NPDB but are not required by law to do so. These include state licensing boards, HMOs, professional societies, and other groups that conduct formal peer review activities.

The NPDB is not currently open to the public. You should be aware, however, that legislation is periodically introduced into Congress to provide public access on at least a limited basis — for example, records of disciplinary action by medical peers or of losses in court of two or more malpractice suits. One Congressional advocate of increased access complains that "Americans are granted more information when purchasing a breakfast cereal than when choosing a heart surgeon." If that view prevails, you may have another important information source at your disposal.

"THE MORE THINGS CHANGE . . ."

Medical knowledge changes rapidly, but so does the organization of medical knowledge. Just as clinical information is increasingly being stored in electronic databases, so are data about hospitals and doctors. Computers not only make it possible to store data; they make it easier to organize them and get access to them. Those who collect and maintain data on health care providers have good reasons for being cautious about releasing some kinds of data to the public, but they are coming under pressure from many places to be somewhat more open. Insurers, for example, have legitimate reasons for wanting statistical data on the track records of hospitals, and hospitals have equally legitimate reasons for wanting to know the track records of doctors. And making data available to any one audience tends to reinforce the claims of others. As more and more institutions (such as insurers, hospitals, and medical societies) insist on fast access to electronic filing cabinets, those who maintain the data in those cabinets often decide that they are better off opening them to everyone under well-publicized rules than trying to justify secrecy or maintain perfect security.

Any movement toward openness will be good news for you. The explosive growth of medical knowledge — and access to it — has given you and your doctor more resources than even the best-trained physicians have ever had before. Even a less-than-explosive growth in access to information about health care providers will improve your ability to hold up your end of a productive partnership with your doctor.

One thing that will not change, however, is the necessity of cultivating that partnership. An earlier chapter notes that what patients need from their doctors is competence and communication. This book has emphasized communication (and its basis in medical knowledge) because it is *your* way of finding and taking advantage of competence. It's hard to overstate this. Although active patients find treatment options their doctors have overlooked often enough to make the effort of searching worthwhile, that's only one reason for becoming an active patient. The *most* important reason is improved communication with your physicians — the key to making sound choices among treatments, facilities, and specialists.

18.

Trust Your Own Judgment

Two doors, or three at most
You think. So should I tell
There may be five or six or more?

I know the door that you should choose
You think. So should I tell
That I sometimes must flip a coin?

One path leads up and one drops down
You think. So should I tell
Up may be down and down around?

I have the map, I know the way
You think. So should I tell
How poor the chart and faint the print?

I'll point the way, you'll follow on
You think. So should I tell
I'll go along and hold your hand?
— "To CM: 55 YO WM w/CAD"
[55-year-old woman with coronary artery disease]
Joseph A. Gascho, M.D.

Physicians generally take great responsibility for the care of their patients. But the practice of medicine holds few certainties, because almost every disease can be treated in one of several different ways, and because individual responses to treatment vary. Thus, the best course of action is not always absolutely clear to doctors.

If they consider the situation carefully — as does Joseph Gascho, who wrote the lines with which this chapter begins — doctors understand that they cannot be infallible and that doctors and patients must work hand in hand to arrive at the best, most healing, choice of treatment. Many physicians welcome a partnership with their patients. Well-informed patients can widen the scope of medical information and improve the decision-making process that so profoundly affects them.

Throughout this book, we have tried to demonstrate some of the means by which you can gain knowledge that will enable you to ask your doctor, and yourself, clear questions and hence increase your chances of finding the most effective medical treatment. The purpose of this chapter is to discuss ways of *applying* your knowledge to benefit you the most.

Evaluating information, discussing it with your primary care physician, consulting with specialists, comparing various options, weighing both objective and subjective considerations, arranging to receive the treatment you want, working with your insurer — all these aspects of reaching your objective will require a pragmatic outlook, leaving preconceived notions behind and letting each experience guide your actions.

A BREAST CANCER PATIENT EXEMPLIFIES PRAGMATISM

The story of Lauren Langford, currently manager of technology for the Community Breast Health Project (described in chapter 8), provides a final example of the importance of trusting your own judgment in the face of a tangle of complex questions and decisions.

For Lauren, the decision process began when a small spot, thought to signal calcification (calcium deposit), showed up on her mammogram. Lauren, then in her early forties and at high risk for breast cancer (with cancer patients on both parents' sides and other risk factors), accepted her radiologist's advice to have an immediate biopsy. Her surgeon recommended a lumpectomy with the biopsy, since the calcification was located deep at the center of the breast, complicating the procedure. That way, he explained, if the calcification proved to be malignant, the cancer would have been removed and a second deeply invasive procedure could be avoided. Lauren agreed and underwent the biopsy-lumpectomy.

The post-surgery pathology report showed the calcification to be nonmalignant but revealed a small, confined carcinoma in a nearby duct — one the surgeon said was "totally independent" of the calcification. He told Lauren that the cancer was located near the margin of the excision he had performed. In cancer surgery, the goal is to remove not a close, but a generous, clear margin of healthy tissue around the suspected cancerous area. Since he didn't have the healthy margin, the surgeon felt there was no way of knowing whether or not there was cancer throughout her breasts. Because of her risk factors, and for symmetry, the surgeon recommended a bilateral mastectomy — complete surgical removal of both breasts.

> I learned this news on a Friday [says Lauren], and I was to go back on Monday to make plans with the surgeon. At first I was stunned by the cancer diagnosis and paralyzed with fear. Then I decided that sitting around wallowing in misery wasn't going to do anybody any good. So my husband and I drove down to the local bookstore and bought all the books we could find that had anything to do with breast cancer. The most useful was *Dr. Susan Love's Breast Book.*

By Monday morning, Lauren had learned from her reading that she had ductal carcinoma in situ (DCIS) and also that calcifications frequently *are* markers for the carcinoma. Could the calcium deposit be a marker for her cancer? Lauren started on a step-by-step process of scrutinizing everything she was told. She asked the surgeon to draw a picture showing how tissue for laboratory slides is dissected and sliced. From his picture, she realized that the block of tissue containing the cancer had not been examined to see if there were calcifications associated with it. She suddenly felt that she was being offered "cookbook medicine" — the one-fits-all standard treatment provided without thought for her individual case. As Lauren puts it,

> I realized that the pathologist had not done a thorough job and that he had simply glossed over my case without giving it any thought. Anger propelled me. And fear was right behind it — the fear of death and the fear that my doctors were not making recommendations based on being fully informed or heavily invested in my situation.

Lauren asked the surgeon to order another test to see if the tissue block containing the cancer also contained any calcification.

She next spent several days at a local university medical library doing literature searches and reading journal articles. She learned that mastectomy was indeed the "gold standard" treatment, but also that recent research on treating DCIS with lumpectomy and radiation was being conducted. She noted that a local researcher, also a pathologist, was one of the world's experts in treating DCIS and had the best record for treating her form of cancer with lumpectomy alone.

At around this time, the first pathologist — after responding to her surgeon's request to reexamine the tissue blocks — had reversed his opinion, saying that the calcification was definitely not a marker for the carcinoma. Lauren had all of her tissue samples and X-rays sent to her new pathologist. The new pathologist carefully studied the samples and noted that although the carcinoma was close to the edges of the excision, a microscopic examination revealed no visible signs of microinvasion of the cancer cells to surrounding tissues. He also concluded that if Lauren had a recurrence of her cancer, it would be marked by calcification.

Gathering confidence as she proceeded with her research and her questions, Lauren finally decided against more extensive surgery. With the report of the second pathologist showing no microinvasion, she believed there was a good chance that her cancer had been completely removed. She would monitor her breasts

closely, especially for calcification, which would warn of any recurrent tumors. In case of a recurrence, she retained the options of
lumpectomy, radiation, or mastectomy.

Her experience left Lauren aware of the importance of being
an active patient:

> I gathered many of the supporting research papers together
> and sent them with a long and detailed cover letter to my in-
> ternist, obstetrician-gynecologist, mammographer, and sur-
> geon, informing them of my decision and explaining my
> reasoning. I told them I needed to be followed carefully for
> three years and asked for their support. All of them agreed to
> support me.
>
> My surgeon still says that he is not happy about my deci-
> sion, but he does follow me closely, and we are able to dis-
> cuss it. My surgeon did a great job. So I have to compliment
> him on his work and also on the fact that he was willing to
> answer any questions I asked along the way and draw pic-
> tures of whatever I wanted to know, and also to direct the
> pathologist to obtain more information from my tissue
> slides.

She also knows that her surgeon was suggesting a standard procedure. "Eighty percent or more of the doctors in the United States
would have recommended the more radical treatment for my situation," Lauren sums up. "It was the 'gold standard,' but it was
not necessarily the best treatment for me."

LESSONS FROM LAUREN'S EXPERIENCE

Does Lauren believe that her doctors were unnecessary in helping
her arrive at a final treatment decision? Is she completely certain
that she made the right medical choice? The answer to both questions is, of course, "no." Lauren recognized that her welfare de-
pended, and still depends, upon her doctors' skills and expertise.
She reconciled herself to differing with their more conservative
approach to her treatment, she found ways of cooperating, and she

in turn gained *their* cooperation. And although Lauren does not pretend to be certain that she made the right medical decision, it was the decision that *seemed* — objectively and subjectively — best to her.

No book could have told Lauren, step by step, how she could best handle her particular situation. She had to learn and improvise as she went along. The only fixed principle was the goal of finding what was for her the best treatment. "The confidence to believe in your own judgment in the face of many opposing viewpoints," says Lauren Langford, "is an absolute necessity."

TRUSTING YOURSELF STILL TAKES GUTS

There will almost always be risks and benefits associated with any choice, and sorting them out may often be difficult. Even after having done your best, you may have doubts.

Nevertheless, once you have made the decision to think independently about treatment choices, you are unlikely ever again to be a passive patient. If your decision process has been based on the best available medical information, an open dialogue with your physicians, and a pragmatic assessment of your treatment options, you will feel confident that no one else could have made a better decision for you.

"Illness," says Susan Sontag in *Illness as Metaphor*, "is the nightside of life, a more onerous citizenship. Sooner or later each of us is obliged, at least for a spell, to identify ourselves as citizens of that other place." Not all the people whose stories have been told in this book have been successful in leaving that other place. Some of them are still living with difficult medical conditions. Not one of them, however, has ever expressed regret about his or her decision to become an active patient and undertake a search for the best treatment.

We admire their determination and courage, and we wish *you* all the luck in the world as you undertake your search.

APPENDIX A

National Network of Libraries of Medicine (NN/LM)

The national network comprises eight regional libraries, each responsible for a geographic area. These libraries coordinate activities within each region and handle requests for health literature not available locally, passing on to NLM requests they cannot fill.

1. MIDDLE ATLANTIC REGION
   The New York Academy of Medicine
   2 East 103rd Street
   New York, New York 10029
   Phone: (212) 876-8763
   Fax: (212) 722-7650
   States served: Delaware, New Jersey, New York, Pennsylvania

2. SOUTHEASTERN/ATLANTIC REGION
   University of Maryland at Baltimore
   Health Sciences Library
   111 South Greene Street
   Baltimore, Maryland 21201
   Phone: (301) 328-2855
   Fax: (301) 328-8403
   States served: Alabama, Florida, Georgia, Maryland, Mississippi, North Carolina, South Carolina, Tennessee, Virginia, West Virginia, District of Columbia, Puerto Rico, U.S. Virgin Islands

3. GREATER MIDWEST REGION
   University of Illinois at Chicago
   Library of the Health Sciences
   P.O. Box 7509

Chicago, Illinois 60680
Phone: (312) 996-2464
Fax: (312) 996-2226
States served: Iowa, Illinois, Indiana, Kentucky, Michigan, Minnesota, North Dakota, Ohio, South Dakota, Wisconsin

4. MIDCONTINENTAL REGION
University of Nebraska Medical Center
McGoogan Library of Medicine
600 South 42nd Street
Omaha, Nebraska 68198-6706
Phone: (402) 559-4326
Fax: (402) 559-5498
States served: Colorado, Kansas, Missouri, Nebraska, Utah, Wyoming

5. SOUTH CENTRAL REGION
Houston Academy of Medicine
Texas Medical Center Library
1133 M.D. Anderson Boulevard
Houston, Texas 77030
Phone: (713) 790-7053
Fax: (713) 790-7052
States served: Arkansas, Louisiana, New Mexico, Oklahoma, Texas

6. PACIFIC NORTHWEST REGION
University of Washington
Health Sciences Center Library, SB-55
Seattle, Washington 98195
Phone: (206) 543-8262
Fax: (206) 543-8066
States served: Alaska, Idaho, Montana, Oregon, Washington

7. PACIFIC SOUTHWEST REGION
University of California at Los Angeles
Louise Darling Biomedical Library
10833 Le Conte Avenue
Los Angeles, California 90024-1798
Phone: (213) 825-1200
Fax: (213) 206-8675
States served: Arizona, California, Hawaii, Nevada, U.S. Territories in the Pacific Basin

8. NEW ENGLAND REGION
   University of Connecticut Health Center
   Lyman Maynard Stowe Library
   263 Farmington Avenue
   Farmington, Connecticut 06034-4003
   Phone: (203) 679-4500
   Fax: (203) 679-4046
   States served: Connecticut, Maine, Massachusetts, New Hampshire,
   Rhode Island, Vermont

Medical Information Search Services

THE FOLLOWING SERVICES, listed alphabetically, either specialize exclusively in health-related searches or do them often. Most offer a range of options, from standardized packages to customized searches. Their prices vary within the broad ranges mentioned in chapter 15. In using this list or any other, you should check with two or three services before making a decision.

ASSOCIATED INFORMATION CONSULTANTS
P.O. Box 8030
Ann Arbor, MI 48107
(313) 996-5553

GEORGIA CONSUMER MEDICAL CENTER INFORMATION SERVICE CENTER
195 Mark Trail
Atlanta, GA 30328
(404) 256-2538

HEALTH INFORMATION NETWORK
4527 Montgomery Drive, Suite E
Santa Rosa, CA 95409
(800) 743-6996

THE HEALTH RESOURCE, INC.
564 Locust St.
Conway, AR 72032
(501) 329-5272

H.E.R.M.E.S. CONSUMER MEDICAL SEARCH
Marina, CA
(800) 484-9863

JOHN E. LEVIS ASSOCIATES
  32945 Indiana
  Livonia, MI 48150-3766
  (313) 422-8029

MED HELP INTERNATIONAL
  6300 N. Wickham Road, Suite 130
  Box 188
  Melbourne, FL 32940-2029
  (407) 253-9048

MEDCETERA
  4515 Merrie Lane
  Bellaire, TX 77401
  (800) 748-6866

MEDSCAN
  189 Riverside Drive
  Johnson City, NY 13790
  (800) MED-8145

PLANETREE HEALTH RESOURCE CENTER
  2040 Webster St.
  San Francisco, CA 94115
  (415) 923-3681

SCHINE-ON-LINE SERVICES
  39 Brinton Ave.
  Providence, RI 02906
  (800) 346-3287; (401) 751-0120

Works Cited

Berkow, Robert, ed. *Merck Manual of Diagnosis and Therapy*, 17th ed. Rahway, N.J.: Merck Research Laboratories, 1992.

Brandon, Alfred N., and Dorothy R. Hill. "Selected List of Books and Journals for the Small Medical Library," *Bulletin of the Medical Library Association* 91(2), April 1993, 141–168.

Braunwald, Eugene, et al., eds. *Harrison's Principles of Internal Medicine*, 11th ed. New York: McGraw-Hill, 1987.

Bridwell, Keith H., and Ronald L. DeWald, eds. *The Textbook of Spinal Surgery*. Philadelphia: Lippincott, 1991.

Burwell, Helen P., and Carolyn N. Hill, eds. *The Burwell Directory of Information Brokers*. Burwell Enterprises, 1990.

"Carotid Endarterectomy — Specific Therapy Based on Pathophysiology" (editorial), *New England Journal of Medicine* 325(7), August 15, 1991, pp. 505–507.

Chiang, Dudee. *Internet for Medical Librarians: A Syllabus Companion; Finding Newspapers and Magazines Online*. Los Angeles: Norris Medical Library, University of Southern California, 1994. (Internet ID: dchiang@hsc.usc.edu)

Covey, Stephen R. *The Seven Habits of Highly Effective People*. New York: Simon and Schuster, 1989.

Delbanco, Thomas L. "Enriching the Doctor-Patient Relationship by

Inviting the Patient's Perspective," *Annals of Internal Medicine* 116(5), March 1992, pp. 414–418.

Dorland, W. A. *Dorland's Illustrated Medical Dictionary*, 27th ed. Philadelphia: Saunders, 1988.

Gilster, Paul. *The Internet Navigator*, 2nd ed. New York: John Wiley and Sons, 1994.

Greenfield, Lazar J., et al., eds. *Surgery: Scientific Principles and Practice*. Philadelphia: Lippincott, 1993.

Guyatt, Gordon H., et al. "Users' Guides to the Medical Literature II: How to Use an Article About Therapy or Prevention," *Journal of the American Medical Association* 270(21), December 1, 1993, pp. 2598–2601.

Harris, Jay R., ed., *Breast Diseases*. Philadelphia: Lippincott, 1991.

Inlander, Charles B. *Take This Book to the Hospital with You: A Consumer Guide to Surviving Your Hospital Stay*, rev. ed. New York: Random House, 1993.

Jacobs, David S., ed. *Laboratory Test Handbook*, 2nd ed. Baltimore: Williams and Wilkins, 1990.

Jaeschke, Roman, et al. "Users' Guides to the Medical Literature III: How to Use an Article About a Diagnostic Test," *Journal of the American Medical Association* 271(5), February 2, 1994, pp. 389–391. John Wiley and Son, 1994.

Kunz, Jeffrey, R. M. Asher, and J. Finkel, eds. *American Medical Association Family Guide*. New York: Random House, 1987.

Larson, David E. *Mayo Clinic Family Health Book*. New York: William Morrow, 1990.

Levine, Mitchell, et al. "Users' Guides to the Medical Literature IV: How to Use an Article About Harm," *Journal of the American Medical Association* 271(20), May 25, 1994, pp. 1615–1619.

Love, Susan M. *Dr. Susan Love's Breast Book*. Reading, Mass.: Addison-Wesley, 1991.

Martindale, William. *The Extra Pharmacopoeia*, 30th revised ed. Edited by James E. F. Reynolds. London: The Pharmaceutical Press, 1993.

Minton, John P. "Results of Surgical Excision of One to 13 Hepatic Metastases in 98 Consecutive Patients," *Archives of Surgery* 124, January 1989, pp. 46–48.

Mosby's Medical, Nursing, and Allied Health Dictionary. St. Louis: Mosby-Year Book, Inc., 1994.

Naifeh, Steven, and Gregory White Smith. *Best Doctors in America*. Aiken, S.C.: Woodward/White, 1994–95.

270 ∎ INFOMEDICINE

National Library of Medicine. *The Basics of Searching MEDLINE: A Guide for the Health Professional.* U.S. Government Printing Office, 1989.

National Library of Medicine. *Cumulated Abridged Index Medicus.* Bethesda, Md.: National Institutes of Health. U.S. Department of Health and Human Services, 1994.

National Library of Medicine. *Cumulated Index Medicus.* Bethesda, Md.: National Institutes of Health. U.S. Department of Health and Human Services, 1994.

National Library of Medicine. *Medical Subject Headings.* Bethesda, Md.: National Institutes of Health. U.S. Department of Health and Human Services, 1994.

National Library of Medicine. *Permuted Medical Subject Headings.* Bethesda, Md.: National Institutes of Health. U.S. Department of Health and Human Services, 1994.

North American Symptomatic Carotid Endarterectomy Trial Collaborators. "Beneficial Effect of Carotid Endarterectomy in Symptomatic Patients with High-Grade Carotid Stenosis," *New England Journal of Medicine* 325(7), August 15, 1991, pp. 445–453.

Norton, Todd, ed. *Transplant Center Access Directory*, 9th ed. Minneapolis, Minn.: National Marrow Donor Program, 1995.

Oxman, Andrew D., et al. "Users' Guides to the Medical Literature I: How to Get Started," *Journal of the American Medical Association* 270(17), November 3, 1993, pp. 2093–2097.

Physicians' Desk Reference. Montvale, N.J.: Medical Economics Production Co., 1994.

Schine, Gary. *If the President Had Cancer . . . : Cancer Care: How to Find and Get the Best There Is.* Providence, R.I.: Sandra Publications, 1993.

Science Citation Index. Philadelphia: Institute for Scientific Information, 1994.

Sontag, Susan. *Illness as Metaphor.* New York: Farrar, Straus and Giroux, 1978.

Stedman's Medical Dictionary, Illustrated, 25th ed. Baltimore: William and Wilkins, 1990.

The Official ABMS Directory of Board Certified Medical Specialists, 26th ed. New Providence, N.J.: Marquis Who's Who, 1994.

Thomas, Clayton L. *Taber's Cyclopedic Medical Dictionary.* Philadelphia: F. A. Davis, 1993.

Webster's Medical Desk Dictionary. Springfield, Mass.: Merriam-Webster, 1986.

White, Barbara J., and Edward J. Madara. *The Self-Help Sourcebook: Finding and Forming Mutual Aid Self-Help Groups*, 5th ed. Denville, N.J.: Northwest Covenant Medical Center, 1995.

Wyngaarden, James et. al., eds. *Cecil Textbook of Medicine.* Philadelphia: Saunders, 1992.

Suggested Readings

This list contains only a small sampling of potentially useful references, both technical and nontechnical, annotated where pertinent.

American Hospital Association Guide to the Health Care Field. Chicago: American Hospital Association, 1994. Probably the most comprehensive listing of hospitals available; with census information, including deaths and births. An in-depth resource that includes information on the following categories: abstract services and indexes; annuals, reviews, and yearbooks; associations and professional societies; bibliographies, directories, and biographical sources; encyclopedias and dictionaries; handbooks and manuals; online databases; periodicals; popular works and patient education; research centers; institutions; clearinghouses; standards; statistics sources; textbooks and general works.

Annas, George J. *The Rights of Patients: The Basic ACLU Guide to Patient Rights*, 2nd ed. Totowa, N.J.: Humana Press, 1992. Written by an attorney who teaches health law at a major university medical school, this book provides a clearly written, objectively stated, and carefully documented overview of its subject.

Bair, Frank E., ed. *The Cancer Sourcebook, vol. 1. Basic Information on Cancer Types, Symptoms, Diagnostic Methods, and Treatments, Including Statistics on Cancer Occurrences Worldwide and the Risks Associated with Known Carcinogens and Activities.* Detroit: Omnigraphics, 1990. Recommended mainly as a ready information source.

Bates, Barbara. *A Guide to Physical Examination and History Taking*, 4th ed. Philadelphia: Lippincott, 1993. Comprehensive description and instruction for medical students. Contains informative and detailed material on the nature and content of the medical examination.

Berczeller, Peter H. *Doctors and Patients: What We Feel About You.* New York: Macmillan, 1994. A physician's incisive, engaging account of the doctor-patient relationship.

Boyden, K., ed. *Medical and Health Information Directory: A Guide to Associations, Agencies, Companies, Institutions, Research Centers, Hospitals, Clinics, Treatment Centers, Educational Programs, Publications, Audiovisuals, Data Banks, Libraries, and Information Services in Clinical Medicine*, 4th ed. 3 vols. Detroit: Gale, 1993. Highly comprehensive directory covering a wide range of medical resources.

Cohen, P. T., Merle A. Sande, and Paul A. Volberding, eds. *The AIDS Knowledge Base: A Textbook on HIV Disease from the University of California, San Francisco, and the San Francisco General Hospital*, 2nd ed. Boston: Little, Brown, 1994. An essential, complete information resource for almost any aspect of HIV. Written for physicians.

Dawson, David M., and Thomas D. Sabin, eds. *Chronic Fatigue Syndrome.* Boston: Little, Brown, 1993. Written for physicians. Contains full information on every facet of this complex syndrome.

Dulbecco, Renato, ed. *Encyclopedia of Human Biology.* San Diego: Academic Press, 1991. Highly informative material relating to the biological basis of medical conditions. Good, primary resource. Technical but easy to follow; excellent organization, with glossaries and references.

DeVita, Vincent, Jr., Samuel Hellman, and Steven A. Rosenberg, eds. *Cancer: Principles and Practice of Oncology*, 3rd ed. Philadelphia: Lippincott, 1989. Impressively comprehensive resource covering the huge subject of cancer, including thorough descriptions of current treatments; written for physicians. Contains excellent references to other literature.

Freed, Melvyn N., and Karen J. Graves. *The Patient's Desk Reference: Where to Find Answers to Medical Questions.* New York: Macmillan,

1994. Well organized. This and Rees (below) are the most comprehensive consumer guides to medical information sources.

Heymann, Jody. *Equal Partners: A Physician's Call for a New Spirit of Medicine.* Boston: Little, Brown, 1995. A physician's memoir of her experience as a seriously ill patient.

Larschan, Edward J. *The Diagnosis Is Cancer: A Psychological and Legal Resource Handbook for Cancer Patients, Their Families and Helping Professionals.* Palo Alto, Calif.: Bull Publishing Co., 1986. Useful, clearly presented work written by a cancer patient who was both a clinical psychologist and an attorney.

Lerner, Max. *Wrestling with the Angel: A Memoir of My Triumph over Illness.* New York: Simon & Schuster, 1990. A famous journalist who became a highly active patient offers a moving and instructive account of his journey to restored health.

Medical Sciences International Who's Who. Detroit: Gale, 1992. If you know the name of the doctor, this is a good resource for a quick look at a physician's credentials here or outside the U.S.

Price, Reynolds. *A Whole New Life.* New York: Macmillan, 1994. A distinguished author's chronicle of how he has actively confronted a debilitating and painful illness.

Rees, Alan M., ed. *The Consumer Health Information Source Book*, 4th ed. Phoenix, Ariz.: Oryx Press, 1994. Excellent popular guide to health information sources and services.

Schwartz, Carol A., and Rebecca L. Turner, eds. *Encyclopedia of Associations*, 29th ed. Detroit: Gale, 1995. This multivolume work contains everything imaginable for networking or information-gathering needs; updated frequently.

Stone, John. *In the Country of Hearts: Journeys in the Art of Medicine.* New York: Bantam, 1992. A series of narratives by a cardiologist who describes what he has learned from his patients about illness and the art of healing.

White, Barbara J., and Edward J. Madara. *The Self-Help Sourcebook: Finding and Forming Mutual Aid Self-Help Groups*, 5th ed. Denville, N.J.: Northwest Covenant Medical Center, 1995. Compact volume offering a good beginning for those interested in self-help groups.

Index

searches, 101, 137–138, 151, 169, 233
See also Grateful Med communications software
MEDNEWS HEALTH INFOCOM Newsletter, 204–205
MEDSIG (Medical Special Interest Group), 146, 178, 179, 202
Mendelsohn, Robert, 18–19
menopause, 183
mental health, 30, 178
Merck Manual of Diagnosis and Therapy, 21, 66–67, 77, 140, 146
mind-body connection, 36–38
Minton, John Peter, 92, 96, 97, 98, 99, 100
miracle cures, 9, 11, 27, 28, 63
modems. *See* computer(s)
Mosaic search tool, 199, 200
Mosby's Medical Dictionary, 64–66
Musella, Al, 24, 26, 189, 237

National Arthritis Foundation, 220
National Cancer Institute (NCI), 144, 175, 203
clinical trials by, 219, 220, 222
National Chronic Pain Outreach Association, 117
National Institutes of Health (NIH), 100, 138, 203, 212
National Kidney Cancer Association (NKCA), 110–11, 150
National Library of Medicine (NLM), 9, 10, 11, 25, 74, 75
accounts, 139–140, 142
databases, 9, 138, 140, 142–144, 153, 194
e-mail address, 139
Index Medicus published by, 79
interlibrary services, 170–171
medical journals index, 76
seminars on searching MEDLARS, 231
See also Grateful Med communications software; MEDLINE
National Marrow Donor Program (NMDP), 110, 111–112
National Multiple Sclerosis Society, 118
National Network of Libraries of Medicine (NN/LM), 75
National Organization for Rare Disorders (NORD), 110, 113–114, 149, 151

National Practitioners Data Bank (NPDB), 254, 255
National Technical Information Service (NTIS), 153
nervous system, 37
New England Journal of Medicine, 17, 76, 102, 215, 253
nonprofit institutions, 140
Northern Lights Alternatives, 182

O'Connor, Sandra Day, 55
Office of Technology Assessment (OTA), 12–13
Official American Board of Medical Specialists (ABMS) Directory of Board Certified Medical Specialists, 71–74, 254
offline planning, 127, 131, 150–151
Ohio State University Medical School, 172, 173
OncoLink database, 177–178, 204
online services, xv–xvi, 25, 136, 233
access to, 135–136, 192–193
active vs. nonactive participation, 185–186
bulletin board service (BBS), 131, 132, 135, 151
charges and fees, 127, 132, 133–134, 135, 139–140, 141, 142, 145, 147, 148, 149, 150, 170, 175, 178–179, 188, 192, 193, 202, 220, 228–230, 233
commercial vendors, 133–135, 140, 145, 179, 192, 193, 194, 200, 203, 205, 206, 230
conference mode sessions, 134–135
defined, 21, 127
discussion groups and forums, 11, 26, 35, 176–178, 190, 193
home pages, 199
institutional accounts, 192, 203, 206
medical searches, 133, 135, 137
messages and message centers, 131–132, 133, 134, 135, 173–174, 177, 178–179, 186–189, 221
message "threads," 147, 174, 176, 181, 204
multiple, 132
people vs. databases, 130–131, 174, 189–190
reference materials on, 133
specialists found through, 57